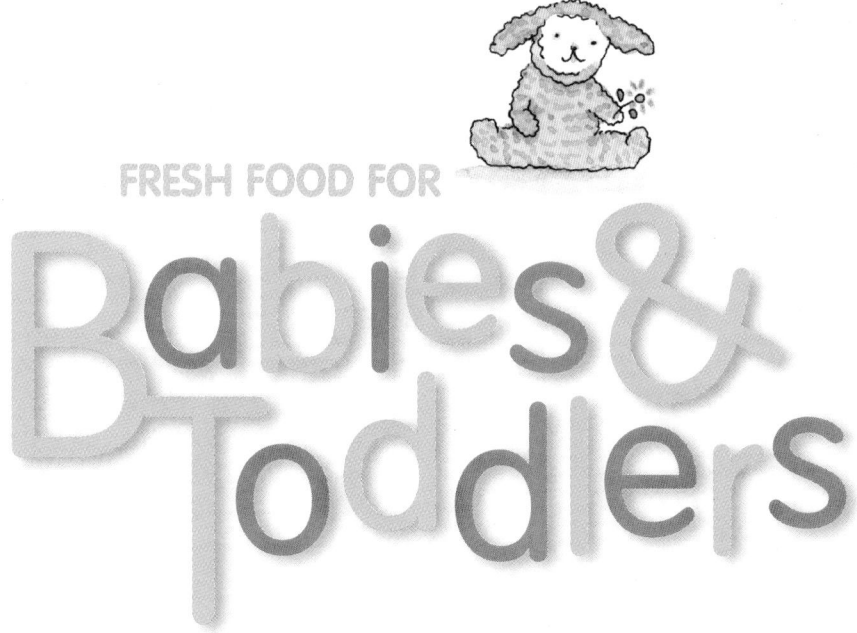

FRESH FOOD FOR

Babies&Toddlers

THE AUSTRALIAN
Women's Weekly

Kids begin developing their eating habits from day one, and that's why it's so important that you start them off on the right foot. Sometimes, deciding what to feed them can be a little confusing, so we've done all the research for you. Here, you'll find more than 100 recipes that are guaranteed to give your kids a good start to a long and healthy life.

Pamela Clark

Food Director

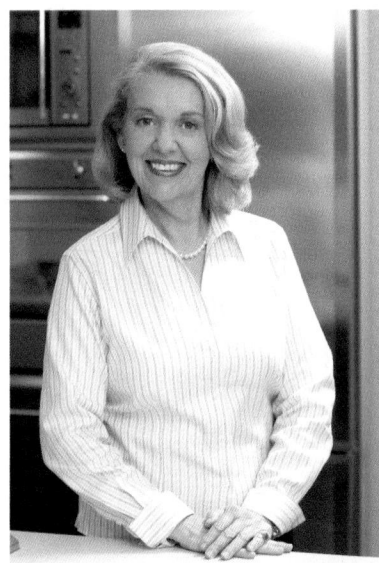

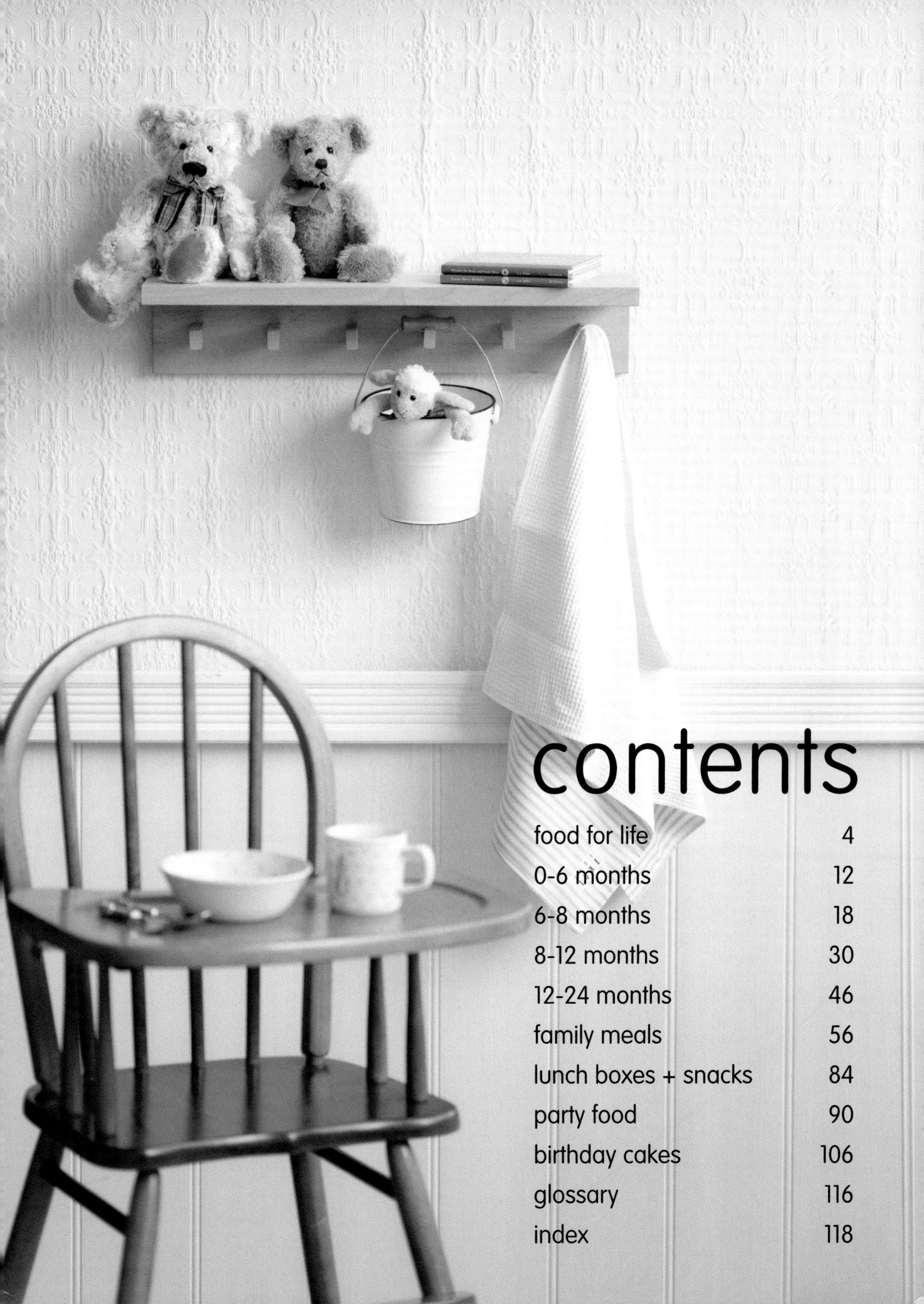

contents

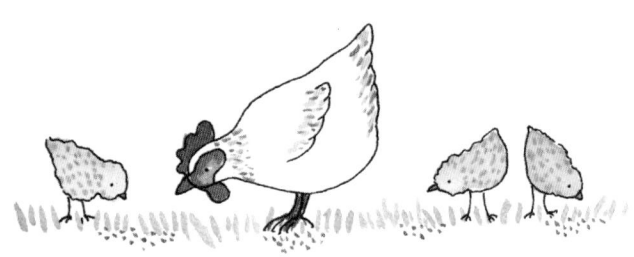

FOOD FOR LIFE

The blessed arrival of a baby is, undeniably, a time of great joy. But look a little closer into the daily function of each newly-formed family, and there's a household in disarray. New parents enter into a learning curve as steep as the south face of Everest. And the area of caring for a baby that gives parents the greatest anxiety is feeding.

Breastmilk or formula? How much? How often? Which bottles to use? How to sterilise bottles? When to introduce solids? What to give? What about fussy eaters? And allergies? Is my baby getting enough?

The questions are endless and there is so much conflicting advice from well-meaning friends and family... Enough!

Trust your instincts

The most important thing to remember is to relax and enjoy parenthood, and the commonsense approach to feeding babies and toddlers adopted in this book should act as reassurance. Under the guidance of a paediatric dietitian, we've compiled a huge number of recipes... recipes for babies' first food, from purées to custards, mashes and mixes for older babies, as well as delicious and well-balanced meals for toddlers of all ages, including a wide variety of dishes that will appeal to the whole family. Our aim is to help you teach your child good food habits, for a long, healthy and active life.

This is also a book to set your mind at ease, not to remind you of all the things you're not doing. A select amount of reading is prudent, to ensure that your child is eating a nutritionally balanced diet, but it's important also to learn to listen to your inner voice when it comes to knowing what's right for your child. Gauge your child's wellbeing by their happy demeanour, regular sleeping patterns and overall good health (including weight gain), not necessarily by the quantity of food that passes their lips. Each and every child is a unique individual, easygoing in some ways and fussy in others, and no child ever comes with a rulebook. Familiarise yourself with the views of the health professionals, but amend their tips and advice to suit your family circumstances and your child. So long as you are always acting out of love for your child, you should be confident that you are the best parent your child could hope for.

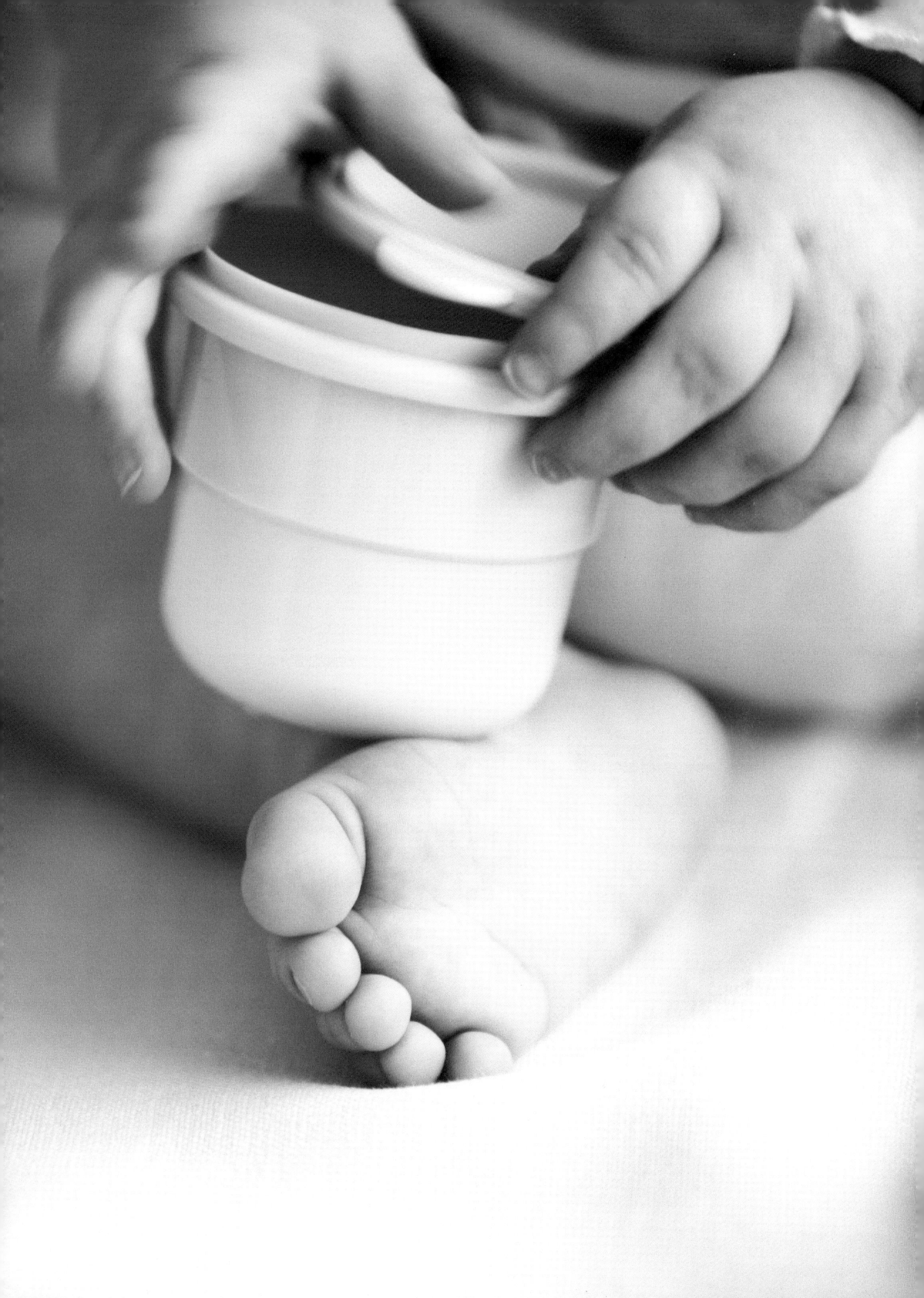

What you'll need

To begin, you will need to purchase a variety of kitchen equipment to make feeding your baby as simple as possible.

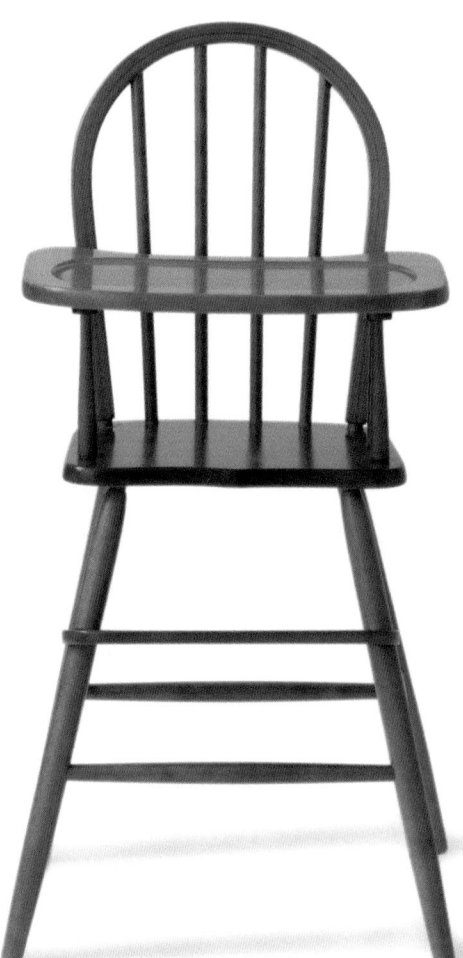

At the most basic level, you should have:

- a selection of bottles (with measurements clearly indicated up the side); if breastfeeding, these are necessary to store expressed breastmilk. If bottle-feeding, you'll need at least six bottles

- teats

- a breast pump (if you are breastfeeding)

- bibs and face washers

- unbreakable plates and bowls

- cups with drinking straws or spouts

- soft-edged spoons

- a fork or potato masher (to mash baby's food)

- a small steaming basket (to fit all saucepan sizes)

- a large saucepan (for sterilising bottles)

- small plastic containers, complete with lids.

Beyond that, it really depends on how much you want to spend and how useful you think you'll find various other pieces of equipment.

Other items you may find useful include:

- potato ricer or mouli
- strainers
- hand-held blender or blender or food processor
- microwaveable bottle steriliser
- high chair (usually not appropriate until baby is at least six months old).

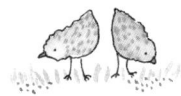

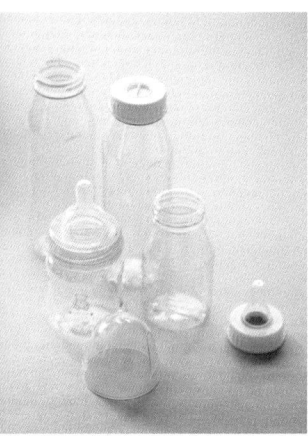

a selection of bottles...

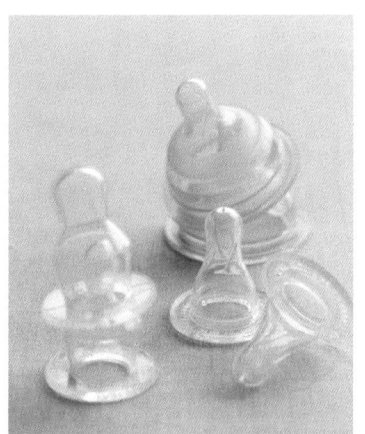

...and teats to fit

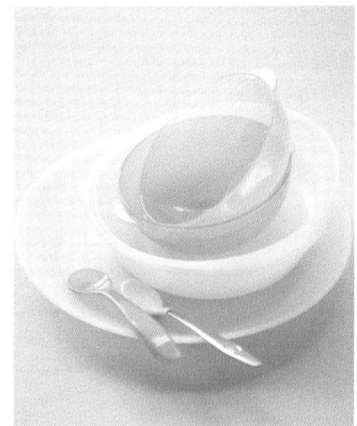

plastic bowls and soft-edged
spoons ensure mealtime safety

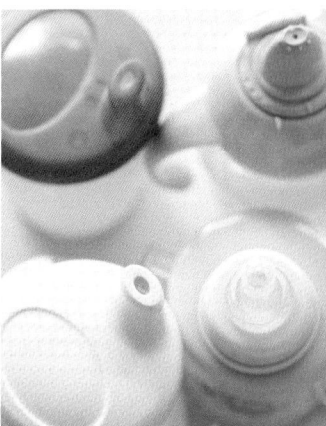

spouted cups can help
reduce spillage

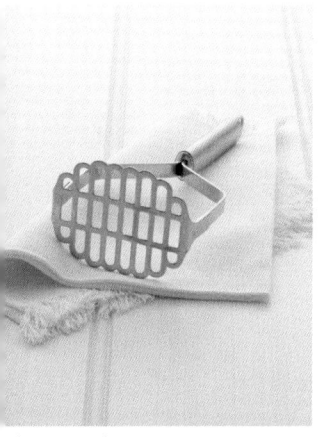

the simplest way to prepare
food is using a masher

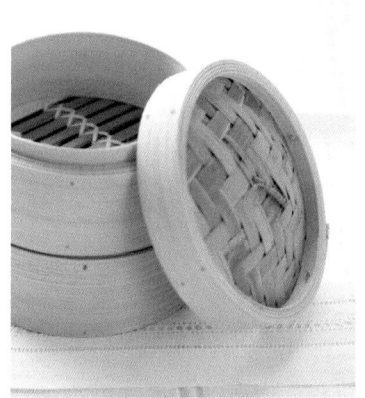

bamboo steamers are ideal
– and inexpensive

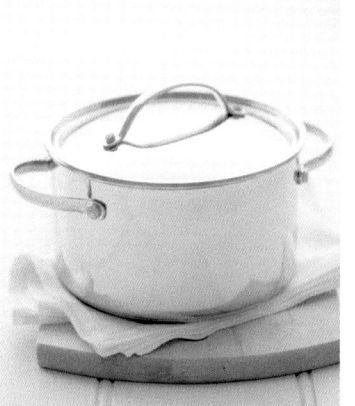

a large saucepan is all that's
required for sterilising

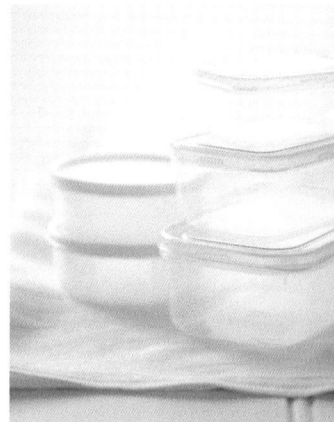

small lidded containers
for freezing and storing

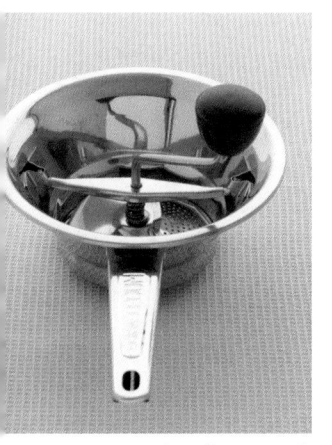

a mouli will turn soft
foods to purée

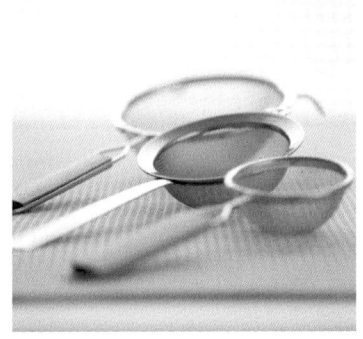

strainers are available
in a variety of sizes

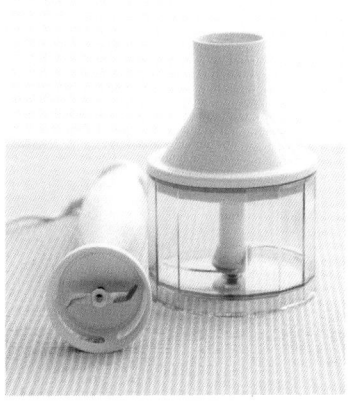

hand-held blenders
can prove useful

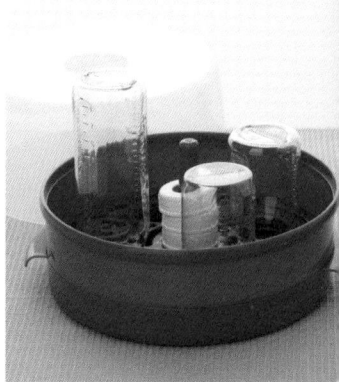

a microwaveable
bottle steriliser

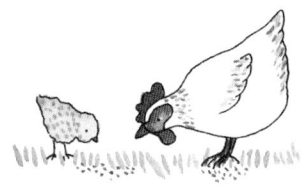

Allergy alert

Thankfully, food allergies are not something most of us need worry about, as less than 10 per cent of children develop true food allergies. More often than not, the babies and toddlers that do develop an allergy have been born into a family with a history of known allergy.

That said, it is still important that when you introduce the most allergenic foods to your baby, you do so under a watchful eye. If there is no family history of allergy and your baby has not been diagnosed with a food allergy, start introducing solids with a low-allergy risk (think rice cereal, fruit and vegetables) around six months of age (see page 18 for how). Take particular care when introducing the most common allergens (see right), giving only a small amount to start with and waiting five to 10 days before introducing another. For instance, anytime after eight months of age is ideal to offer your baby a small amount of egg yolk; if you observe no reaction, you can then offer the more allergenic egg white.

Common allergens

The most common allergens are eggs, peanuts and milk; reactions have also occurred after consumption of fish/seafood, soy beans and other legumes, other nuts, sesame seeds and wheat.

Allergies to food can cause a range of symptoms. Some symptoms can follow immediately after consumption, and include swelling of the lips and a red rash around the mouth. This can be accompanied by vomiting, diarrhoea, stomach pains or a rash elsewhere on the body. (In some cases – but not all – eczema may be food related.) In the event of a severe allergic reaction, symptoms can include a tightness in the throat or chest, difficulty breathing or swallowing and even a loss of consciousness.

It is obvious then, that correct diagnosis of a food allergy is important, so that your child is not exposed to foods that could make him ill or limited unnecessarily from consuming certain foods. The good news, though, is that young children often grow out of food allergies, though reactions to peanuts, other nuts and fish tend to persist.

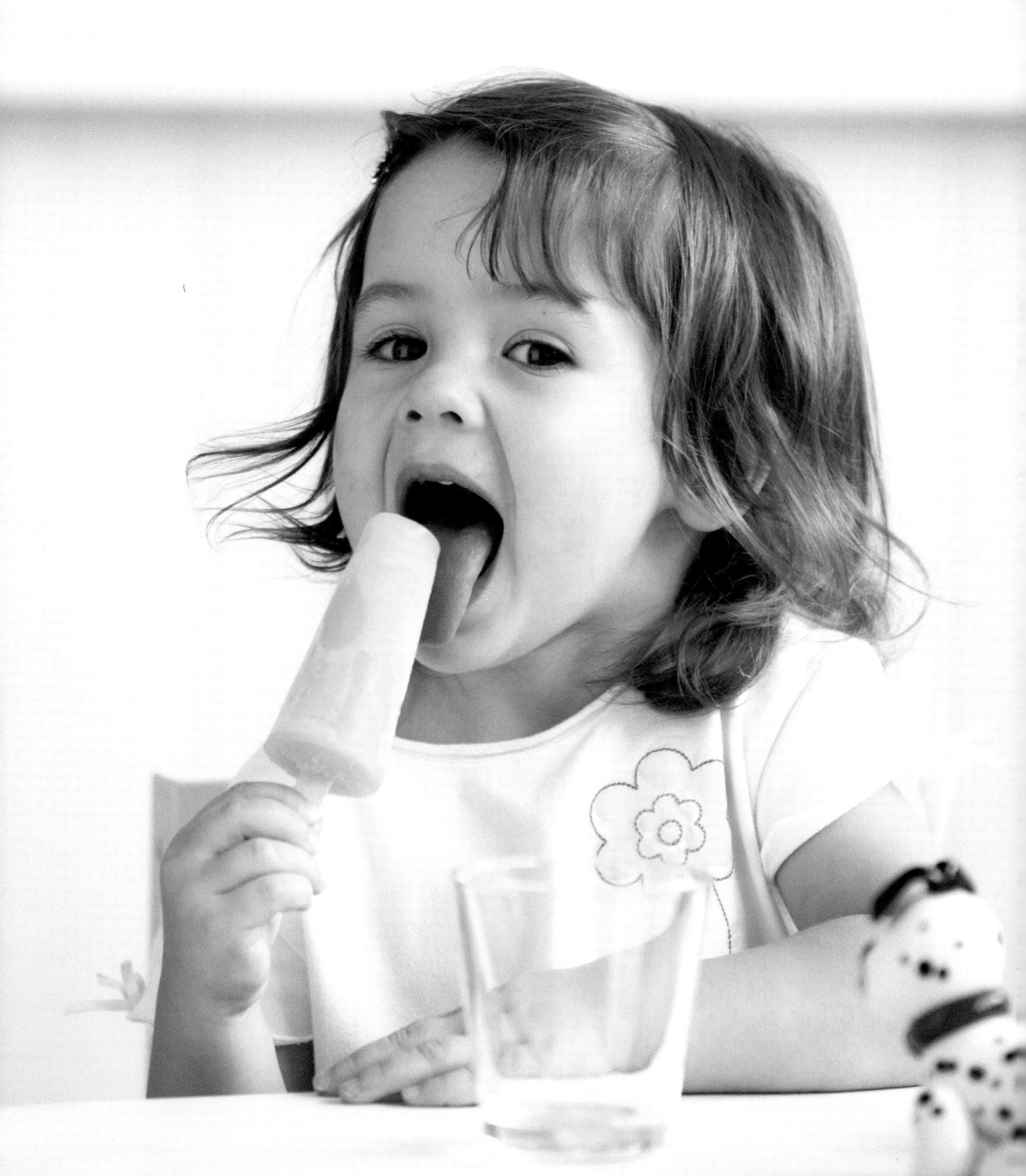

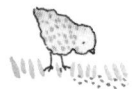

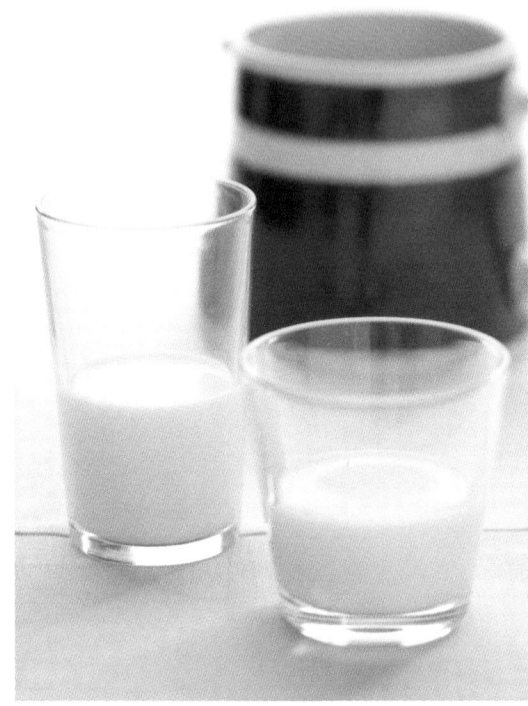

Milk-feeding allergic babies

While breastfeeding is the best way to feed your baby if there is a history of known allergy in your family, you should be aware that allergens can pass through breastmilk. Avoidance of common food allergens in the mother's diet may be recommended if your baby is diagnosed with an allergy. It is far less clear whether avoidance of allergens while breastfeeding can actually prevent

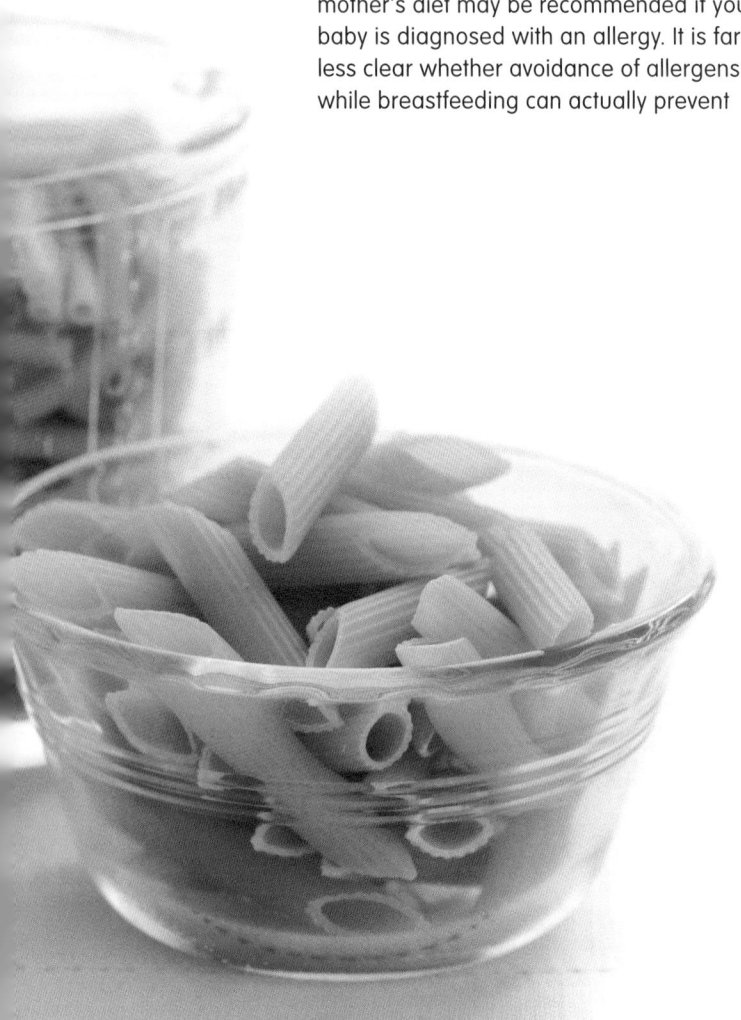

an allergy in your baby. It is important to recognise, too, that if you cut milk from your diet, for example, you risk nutritional imbalance. That said, if the allergen in your family is peanuts, there is a case for cutting all peanut sources from your diet while you are breastfeeding. Make an appointment with your doctor to discuss your options and see an accredited dietitian if food restrictions are recommended.

If you are not breastfeeding and have a strong family history of allergy, it could be a good idea to choose an infant formula in which the cow's milk protein has been partially broken down. These formulas usually contain the letters "HA" in their name – ask your pharmacist for help. These formulas may not be suitable, however, for those babies with a diagnosed cow's milk allergy. In the case of a milk allergy, your doctor will be able to recommend a suitable formula for your child, depending on their symptoms.

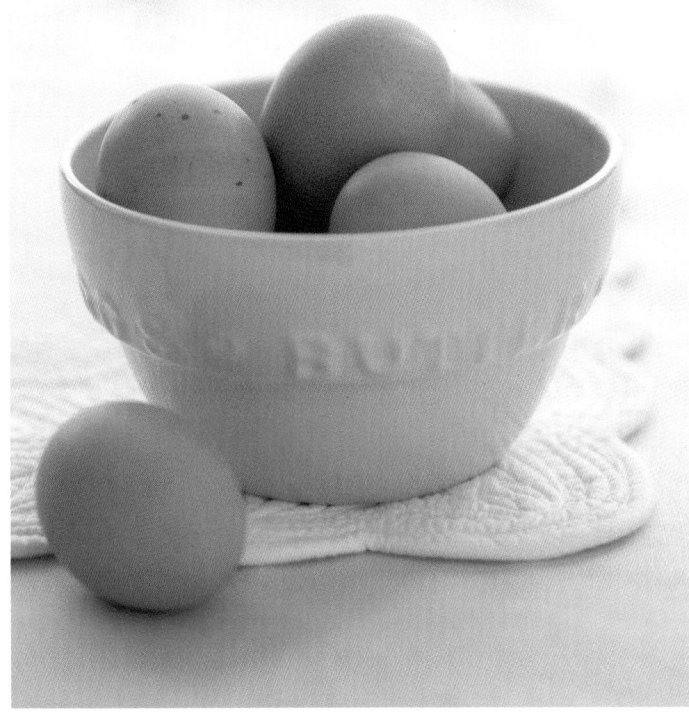

Food for children who are allergic

The immune system is quite immature in the first year of a baby's life so, for those babies at risk of food allergies, it is important not to introduce food too early. Hold back on introducing solids to your baby until they are six months old.

If your baby has been diagnosed with specific food allergies, they must not be fed any food that contains any trace of that allergen. You should be advised by your doctor as to when other food allergens can be introduced. As a general rule, however, don't offer known allergens such as milk and other dairy products (including cheese, yogurt, ice-cream, etc), peanuts and other nuts, wheat and soy products, eggs and fish, and all products that contain any of these allergens, until your child is 12 months of age.

When you do introduce these foods, offer only small amounts to begin with and wait for five to 10 days before introducing another known allergen.

The parents of children with food allergies need to become vigilant food-label readers, as there are a multiplicity of foods that may contain the allergen that is a threat to your child's health. Referral to an accredited practising dietitian can help you find these hidden sources and come up with alternative foods. It is also imperative that you teach your child from a very young age about the foods they must not eat, and ensure that grandparents, day-care or pre-school staff, and all other adults that come into contact with your child are reliably informed about the allergy and what to do in the event of an allergic reaction. Your GP can teach you the most appropriate way to treat your child's particular allergic reaction.

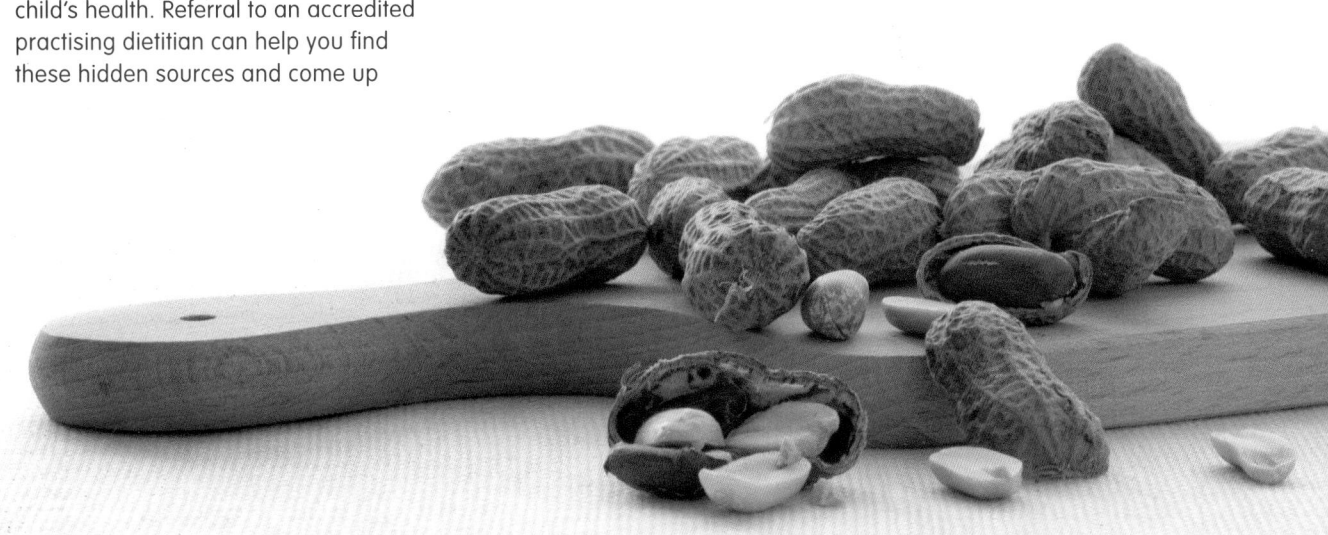

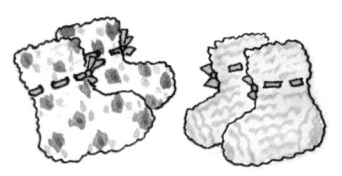

0-6 MONTHS

For the first six months, feeding your baby is all about milk, milk, milk. For time-stretched new parents, it could come as a relief to find there's no cooking required. Read on for tips about bottle sterilisation, breastfeeding, formula feeding and weaning.

Mother's milk

Breastmilk contains a complete balance of nutrients – just what nature intended for newborns. Combine this with the fact that it is stored in germ-free containers – always at the ready – at exactly the right temperature, and it would have to be any mother's first choice, wherever possible.

Once established, breastfeeding is often a tender, sharing experience for mothers and babies. But getting it right – or knowing that you are doing it correctly – can be hard, particularly in the early weeks. There are a number of places from which you can seek expert help: hospitals often employ a lactation consultant or midwife exclusively to help new mums with breastfeeding issues, or visit your local early childhood centre or breastfeeding association. Reassurance and tips about technique can make a world of difference.

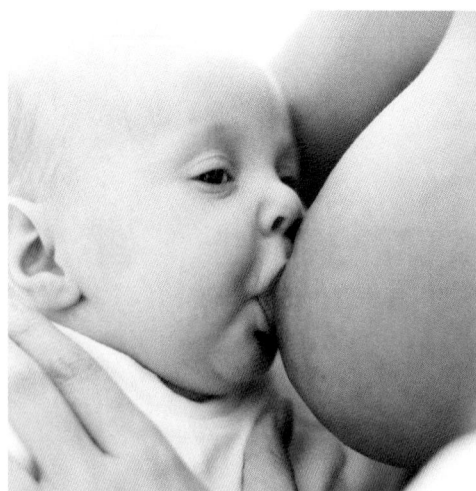

If circumstances have dictated that breastfeeding is not an option, however, don't despair. Today's infant formulas are a close match to breastmilk, so bottle-feeding will meet all of your baby's nutritional needs. Focus on establishing the delightful bonds of intimacy between yourself and your child as you develop their feeding pattern. Get comfortable – settle into the same chair in the same room for each feed – then snuggle in and start to get to know your baby, whether the feed has come from bottle or breast.

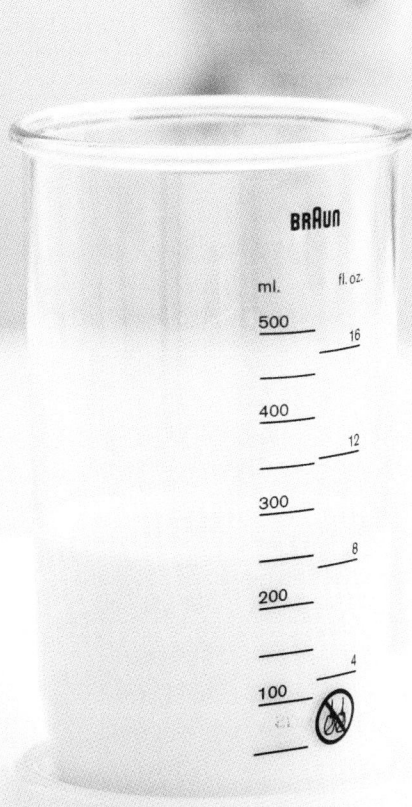
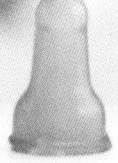

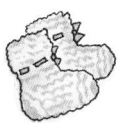

Food for new mothers

Often, in the first chaotic months of motherhood, new mums are inclined to pay far less attention to their own diet than they should. In their overwhelming desire to see that their baby is fed well, and that all of baby's other needs are met, women place themselves at the bottom of their own list of priorities.

But what new mums need to consider is that, while ever they are not eating an adequate amount of nutritionally sound food, they are operating at less than an optimum level.

The lesson here? The best thing you can do for your baby is to look after yourself.

Consider the following:

- Birth may be a natural function, but it is still a physical trauma that your body will take many months to recover from. Your body needs appropriate nourishment to regenerate.

- If you are breastfeeding, you're likely to feel hungry all the time. Don't panic – breastfeeding uses up a lot of energy.

If you're ravenous, eat more – with a focus on fruit, vegetables, bread and cereals, reduced-fat dairy products and lean meat, chicken or fish.

- Avoid actively dieting to lose the weight gained in pregnancy. Your body needs more energy, not less, to produce breastmilk. Be reassured… breastfeeding will help get you back into shape faster.

- Breastfeeding mums will undoubtedly feel thirsty far more often than usual. Answer your body's call – drink some water every time you feed your baby, and have other fluids as you feel the need.

- If you don't eat animal products, make sure you take a vitamin B12 supplement when breastfeeding, so that your baby gets enough of this essential vitamin.

- Ignore the myths about a mother's diet affecting breastmilk supply – sucking at the breast is the stimulus for milk supply. Some breastfeeding mothers report that after having certain foods – typically cabbage, broccoli, brussels sprouts and onions, or large quantities of drink containing caffeine – their babies suffer from general upset. Cut these foods from your diet if you feel your child is reacting to their presence in your milk, and consume no more than three cups of cola or coffee a day. Despite what you may have heard, cutting milk from your diet is unlikely to improve colic symptoms in your baby, and dairy products are an important source of calcium for breastfeeding mums.

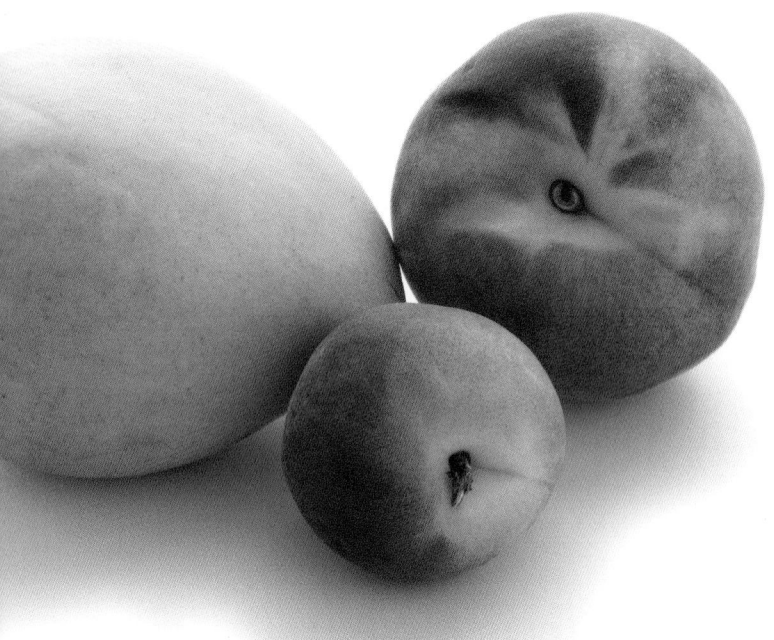

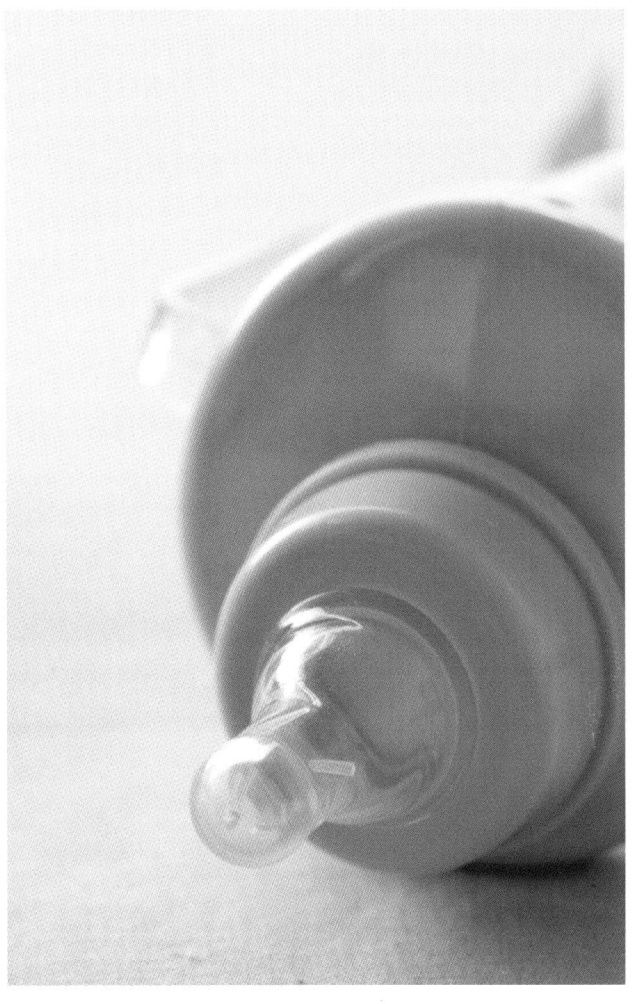

Sterilising equipment

Disinfecting your baby's bottle-feeding equipment (and dummies) is most important in the first 12 months of their life, while their immune system is still immature. A high standard of hygiene can also be achieved by washing your hands carefully before feeds (whether breast or bottle) and after every nappy change.

It's also important to note that all bottles, teats, dummies, etc, should be rinsed in cold water as soon as they are finished with, then washed in hot soapy water (whenever convenient) before being disinfected. Any method you use to disinfect bottles is unlikely to do much if dried old milk remains on bottles or teats.

Any of the following methods can be used to disinfect your baby's equipment...

Boiling water

Dummies, bottles and teats should be boiled for 5 minutes in a large saucepan of water. Allow the equipment to cool in the water until it is able to be handled. Any equipment that's not being used immediately can be stored in a clean container in the fridge, but any unused clean equipment should be re-sterilised every 24 hours or so.

Chemical solutions

Chemical sterilants come in tablet or liquid form; when added to water following the manufacturer's instructions, they form a solution that is dilute enough to be perfectly safe for babies and yet, at the same time, kill the bacteria on your baby's equipment. The bottles, etc, are merely left to soak in the solution for a specified time or until required; however, a new batch of solution needs to be made every 24 hours. One important thing to note when using these chemicals is that the solution will corrode metals, so be sure to only use it with equipment made from plastic or glass.

Steam or microwave sterilisers

Steam and microwave sterilisers can be purchased from baby goods stores; both use steam to disinfect bottles, etc. Both forms of steriliser should be used according to manufacturer's instructions; a microwave steriliser (a lidded plastic container designed to hold bottles) is the less expensive option as a steam steriliser is an electrical appliance.

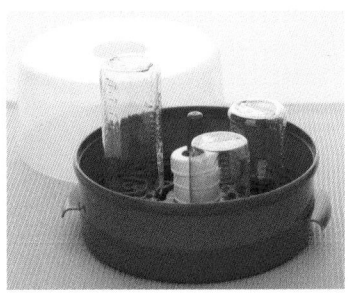

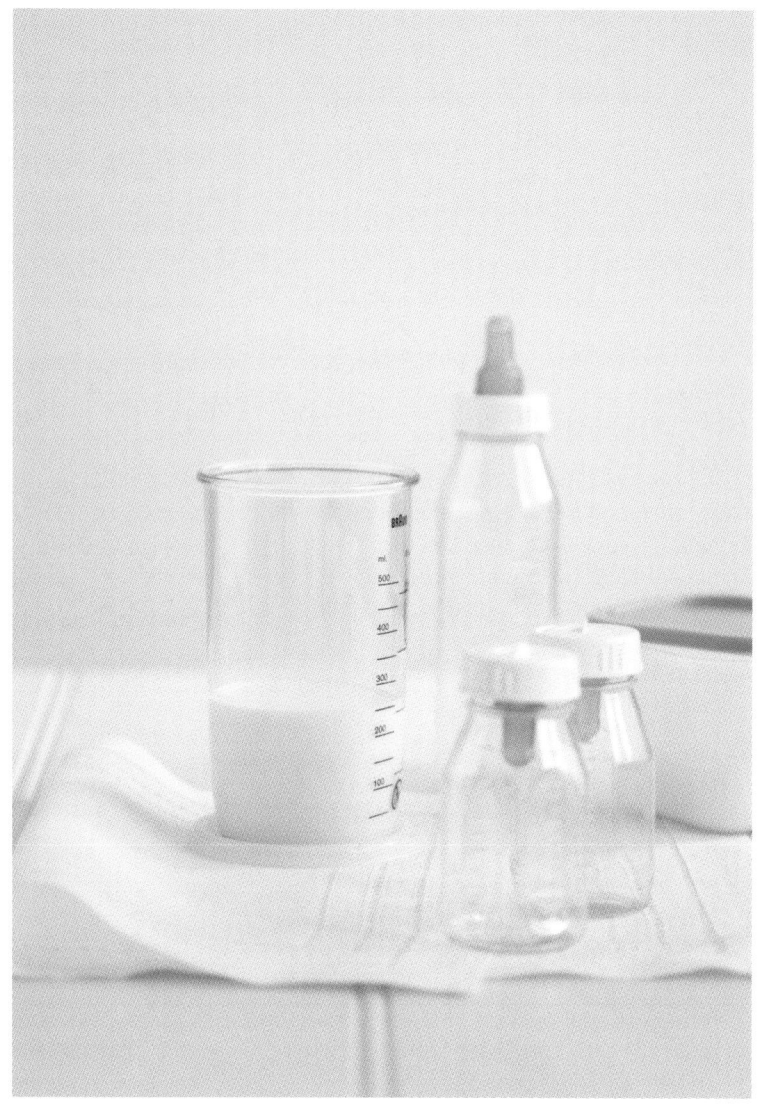

IS MY BABY THE RIGHT WEIGHT?

Unless you have a bonny baby that tips the scales, it's very common as a first-time parent to wonder if your child is eating enough and gaining height and weight as they should. If your baby is happy, healthy, and eating and sleeping well, you should feel reasonably secure in the knowledge that you're doing alright!

Babies vary in size and shape, just like adults. Some appear plump, but that's not to say that they are overweight. Others are small and lean, but that's not to say they are too thin.

Regular visits to your local Early Childhood Centre or GP are the ideal occasion to plot your child's growth on a percentile chart. Any excessive weight gains (or losses) can be measured this way, and your health professional can reassure you that your baby's weight is in proportion to his height.

Selecting an infant formula

Despite what the manufacturers may claim, all infant formulas are basically similar and have to meet strict government standards. The differences between brands are mainly in the added "extras" and, in the main, the jury is still out as to whether these "extras" are of significant benefit. When choosing a formula, you might prefer a specific brand or be influenced by cost or availability, or even how the formula is packaged – only some formulas are available in sachets (as well as the standard large can), making them most suitable for use when travelling or on the odd occasion as a top-up after breastfeeding.

Formulas labelled "from birth" are suitable for newborns up to the age of 12 months. "Follow on" formulas are designed for babies from six months of age and upwards, and should not be used for younger babies. Once you have chosen a formula, stick with it – different formulas may taste different, leading to rejection by your baby.

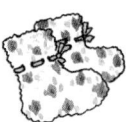

Weaning from the breast

Weaning your baby means that you stop breastfeeding and replace these feeds with other liquids (and solids, depending on your baby's age). The time to wean is when it feels right for you and your baby – or when circumstances make it necessary. If the decision to wean is made reluctantly (perhaps you need to return to work) or breastfeeding just hasn't worked for you, you may feel some sadness. Consider the possibility of combining breastfeeding and formula-feeding – perhaps this might allow you to continue breastfeeding for longer. If this doesn't work and weaning is necessary, don't dismiss your feelings – it's normal to have a bit of a cry. Talking about it with your partner, a friend or an early childhood nurse will help you come to grips with your emotions.

The how-to of weaning depends on the abundance of your milk supply; the aim is to reduce your supply gradually, to avoid the onset of mastitis (red swollen breasts and flu-like symptoms brought on by a bacterial infection). It can take only days to wean if your milk supply wasn't well established (or your older baby isn't a frequent feeder), but plan on it taking four to five weeks. To begin, skip one feed a day, instead giving your baby formula. Continue breastfeeding for the other feeds. Initially, after a missed breastfeed, your breasts will probably feel engorged (you may need to express a little milk for comfort), but this will abate as your body adjusts to the reduced demand. Once your breasts are feeling comfortable (this could take up to a week), drop another daily breastfeed, again replacing it with a formula feed, and so on until weaning is complete. Avoid dropping consecutive feeds, to prevent your breasts from becoming too engorged. As your milk supply shuts down, you may need to offer top-up formula feeds after your remaining breastfeeds, as you may not be producing enough milk for your baby.

DID YOU KNOW?

One benefit of breastfeeding is that breastfed babies are less likely to be overweight children.

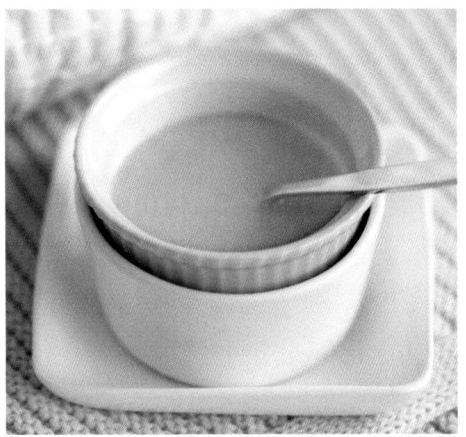

When to feed solids

Breastmilk or formula is all that a baby needs for sustenance and growth in the first six months or so of life. So, around six months of age is a good time to introduce other foods to their diet; anytime before four months of age is too early. The decision to introduce your baby to solids is one that should only be made by you, dependent on your baby's readiness. You may find that well-meaning relatives make suggestions on the subject… that perhaps a baby as big as yours will only sleep through the night if you start him on solids, or maybe that offering solids will prevent your baby's reflux vomiting, or that the way your child chews his fists is a sure indication of his hunger for more than milk. Be assured – there is no accuracy to any of these assertions. Every baby is born with the "extrusion reflex", which means that if you put something to your baby's mouth, his tongue will poke out. This enables babies to effectively suck on the nipple or teat that supplies their milk. If a baby hasn't outgrown this reflex and you try to feed him solids, his tongue will push the food from his mouth, leading you to believe that he won't eat solid food when the case is more that he can't.

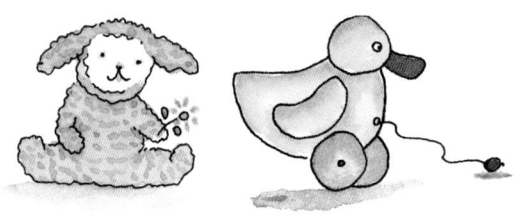

6-8 MONTHS

"Mealtime" has a whole new meaning at this stage of your baby's dietary development; solid foods are now firmly on the agenda. As well as helpful advice, this chapter features innumerable variations on a purée theme – all perfectly delicious baby food.

Introducing solids

When it comes to starting your baby on solids, keep it simple and begin with only tiny quantities. Mix a little rice cereal (purchased from the supermarket) with formula, breastmilk or cooled, boiled water until the blend is quite runny, remembering that your baby is only accustomed to liquids. Feed your baby half a teaspoon or so of the mixture after their milk feed. The next day, offer just a tiny bit more, and gradually increase the amount in the following days until baby is eating 2 tablespoons of rice cereal. When these feeds are running smoothly, start introducing finely mashed or puréed vegetables or fruit in much the same way – beginning with tiny quantities and working up to larger amounts. When introducing new foods, observe your baby closely for signs of a reaction or allergy. And don't interpret your child's refusal of a certain food as a sign that they don't like it. Research has shown that babies opt for familiar foods, so offer your baby a new food up to 10 times before concluding that they don't like it. This can, of course, prove frustrating, but keep your manner calm and measured so your baby doesn't associate feed times with negative feelings.

UNSUITABLE FOODS FOR BABIES

On top of the most common food allergens (see page 8), there are some other edibles that shouldn't be given to babies.
Obvious choking hazards, such as whole raw carrot, celery and apple, corn chips, popcorn, lumps of sausage, hard lollies and whole nuts should be avoided at all costs, though it is worth noting that hard fruits and vegetables can safely be served grated or steamed until soft. Honey is also a no-no for babies under 12 months of age, as it has been known to cause botulism (a type of poisoning).

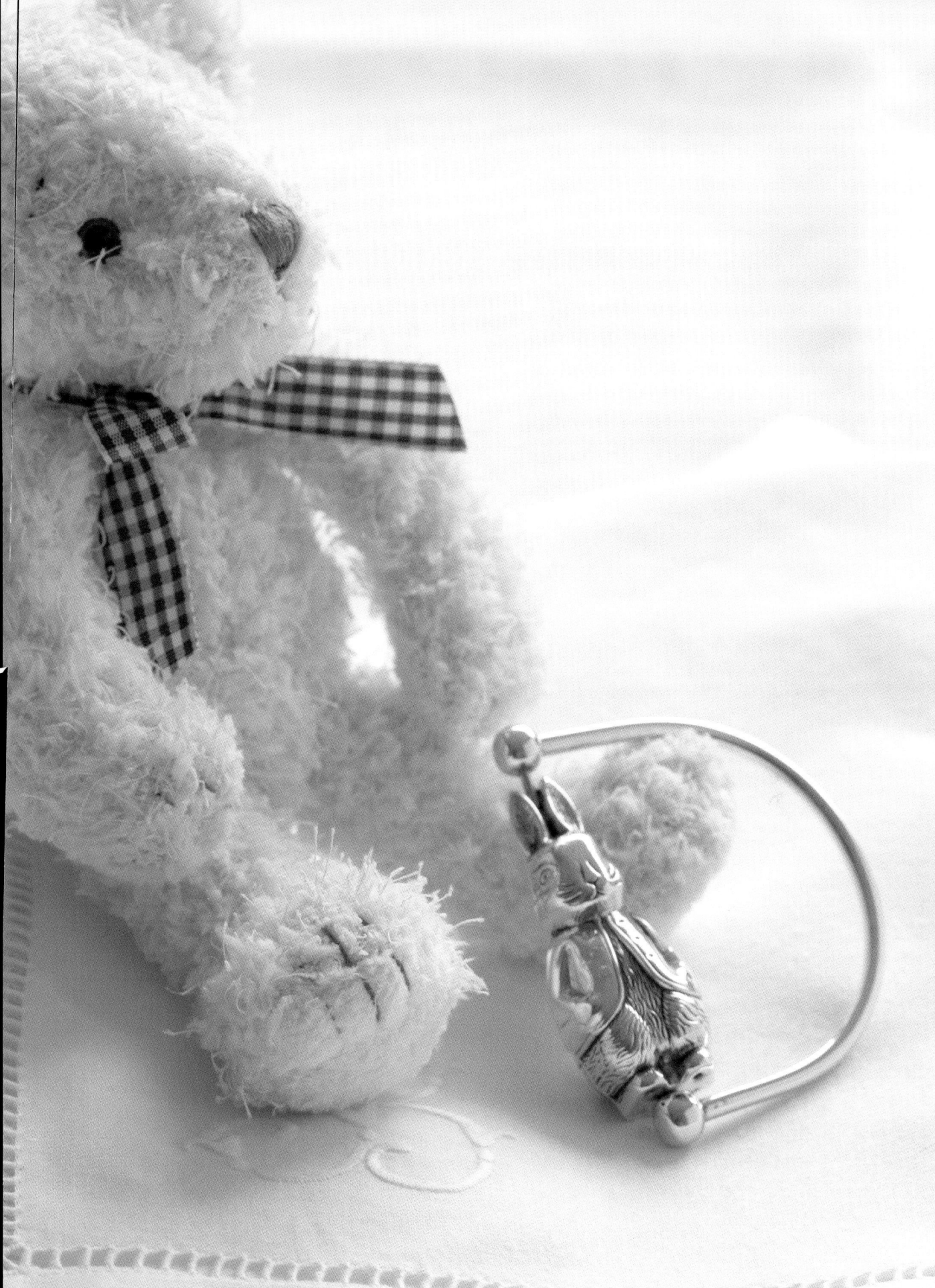

PUREES MADE EASY

The tables on these two pages have been created so you can quickly and easily make your purée of choice, according to the groupings of fruit or vegetable. Read down the first column on the left of each table to find your ingredient of choice, then read across to discover the quantity you'll need, the preparation technique and the time it will take to cook. For a purée that could be slightly gluggy, we've also suggested what quantity of liquid you'll need to add to make it easier for your baby to manage.

fruit purées

ALL PUREES MAKE 1 CUP
(12 TABLESPOONS)

For apple and pear:

1 Combine fruit and the water in medium saucepan; bring to a boil. Reduce heat; simmer, uncovered, until tender.

2 Blend or process fruit mixture until smooth. Give your child as much fruit purée as desired.

For remaining fruit:

Blend or process fruit until smooth. Give your child as much fruit purée as desired.

TIP Fruit and vegetable purées can be frozen in 1-tablespoon batches in ice-cube trays, covered, for up to 1 month.

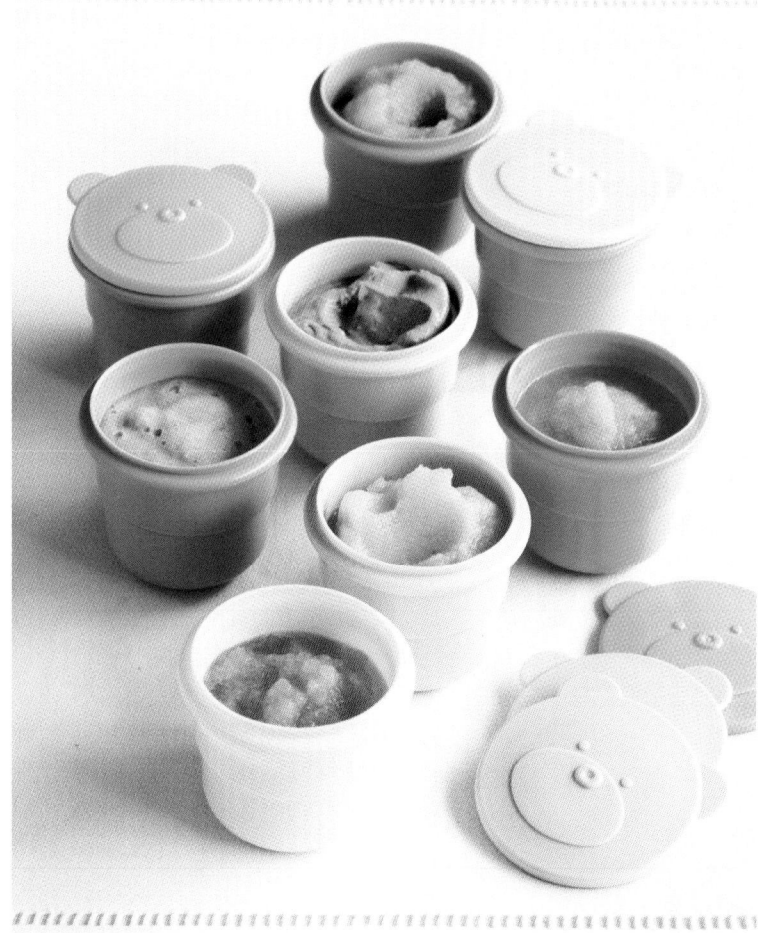

FRUIT	QUANTITY	PREPARATION	COOKING TIME	WATER
Apple	2 large (400g)	Peel, core, chop coarsely	10 minutes	2 tablespoons
Avocado	2 small (400g)	Peel, seed, chop coarsely	-	-
Banana	2 medium (400g)	Peel, chop coarsely	-	-
Custard apple	400g	Peel, seed, chop coarsely	-	-
Pear	1 large (330g)	Peel, core, chop coarsely	20 minutes	2 tablespoons
Rockmelon	500g	Peel (remove all green sections), seed, chop coarsely	-	-

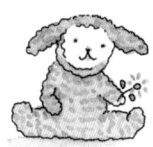

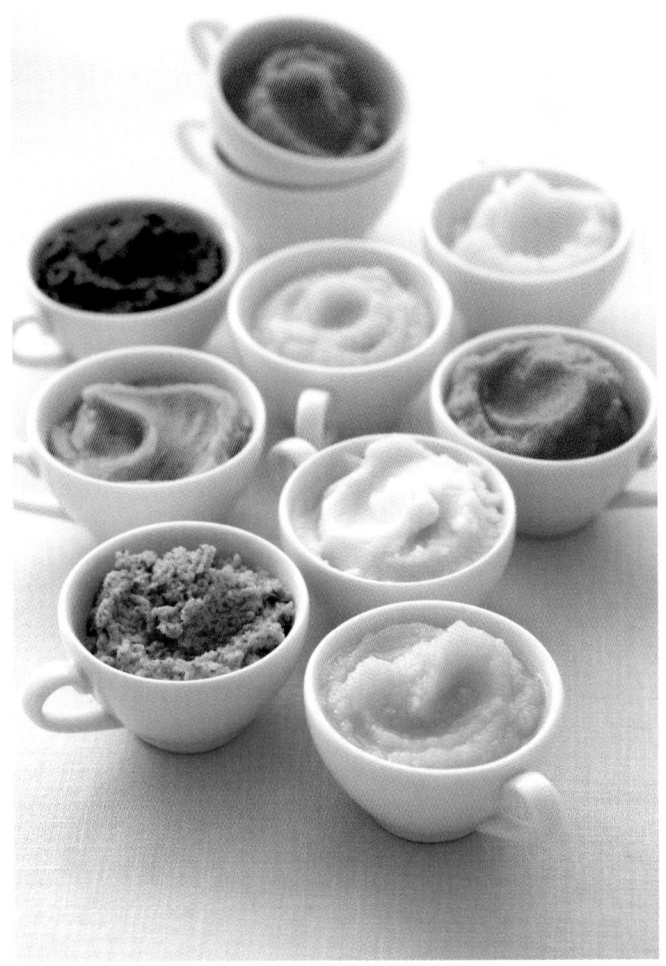

vegetable purées

ALL PUREES MAKE 1 CUP (12 TABLESPOONS)

When puréeing vegetables, you can add breastmilk, formula or water to achieve desired consistency.

For potato and pumpkin:
1 Steam vegetable until tender; drain.
2 Push vegetable through sieve.

For remaining vegetables:
Steam vegetable until tender; drain. Blend or process vegetable (and liquid) of choice until smooth. Give your child as much vegetable purée as desired.

VEGETABLE	QUANTITY	PREPARATION	COOKING TIME	LIQUID
Broccoli	250g	Cut into florets, chop stem coarsely	8 minutes	2 tablespoons
Carrot	2 large (360g)	Trim ends, peel, chop coarsely	15 minutes	2 tablespoons
Cauliflower	250g	Trim stem, cut into florets	8 minutes	-
Kumara	1 medium (400g)	Peel, chop coarsely	20 minutes	1 tablespoon
Potato	2 medium (400g)	Peel, chop coarsely	20 minutes	2 tablespoons
Pumpkin	400g	Peel, remove seeds, chop coarsely	12 minutes	-
Spinach	250g	Trim stems, chop coarsely	8 minutes	1 tablespoon
Patty-pan squash	300g	Trim ends, chop coarsely	12 minutes	-
Zucchini	2 large (300g)	Trim ends, peel, chop coarsely	7 minutes	-

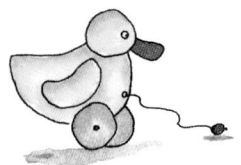

purée combinations

ALL COMBINATIONS MAKE ¼ CUP (3 TABLESPOONS)

All of the purée combinations on these pages are made using the completed fruit and vegetable purées that feature on the previous pages (20-21).

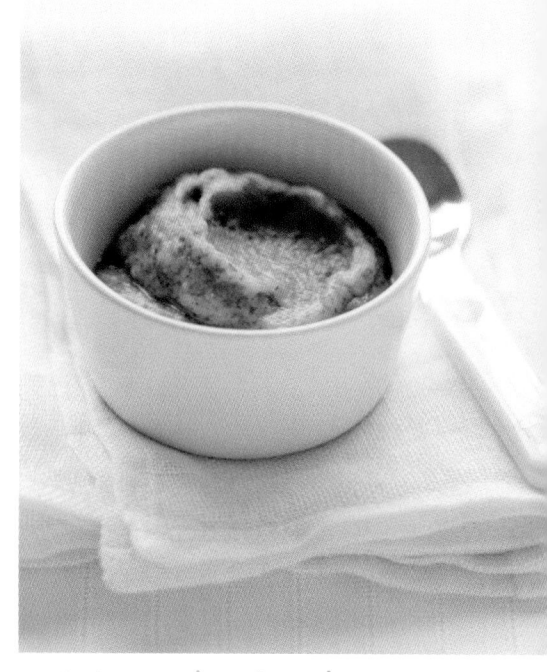

potato and pumpkin

Combine 2 tablespoons puréed potato with 1 tablespoon puréed pumpkin.

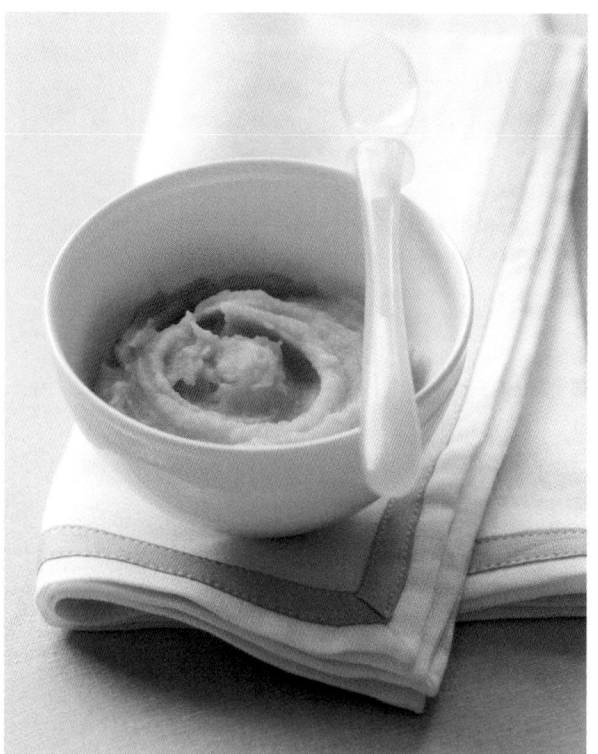

potato and spinach

Combine 2 tablespoons puréed potato with 1 tablespoon puréed spinach.

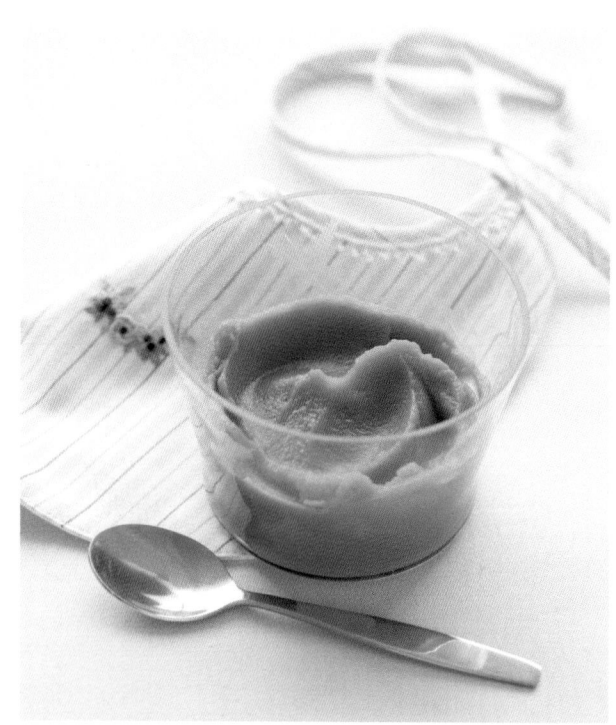

kumara and squash

Combine 2 tablespoons puréed kumara with 1 tablespoon puréed squash.

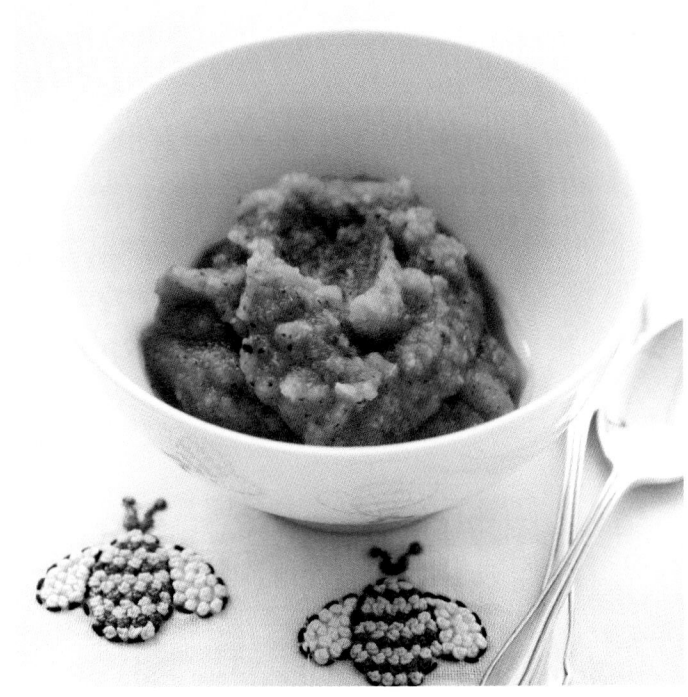

carrot and broccoli

Combine 2 tablespoons
puréed carrot with 1 tablespoon
puréed broccoli.

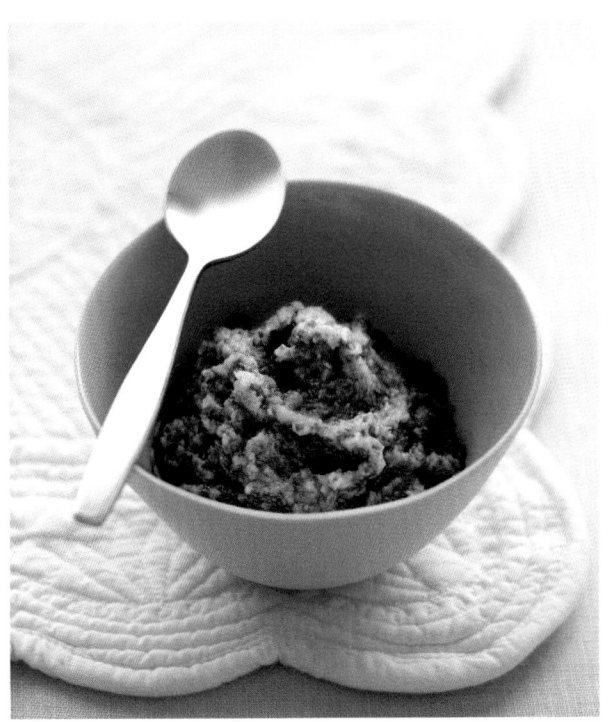

carrot and spinach

Combine 2 tablespoons puréed carrot
with 1 tablespoon puréed spinach.

apple and avocado

Combine 2 tablespoons puréed apple
with 1 tablespoon puréed avocado.

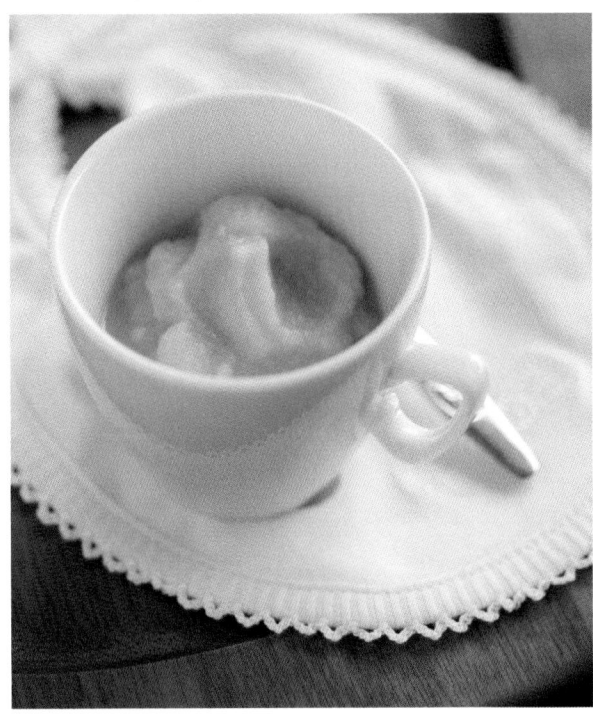

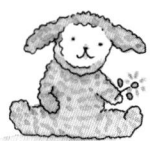

chicken, zucchini and parsnip purée

PREPARATION TIME **10 MINUTES** COOKING TIME **20 MINUTES** MAKES **2 CUPS**

1 single chicken breast fillet (170g),
chopped coarsely

2 small zucchini (180g),
chopped coarsely

1 small parsnip (120g),
chopped coarsely

1¼ cups (310ml) water

1 Place ingredients in small
saucepan; bring to a boil.
Boil, uncovered, until
vegetables soften and
chicken is cooked through.

2 Blend or process mixture
until smooth.

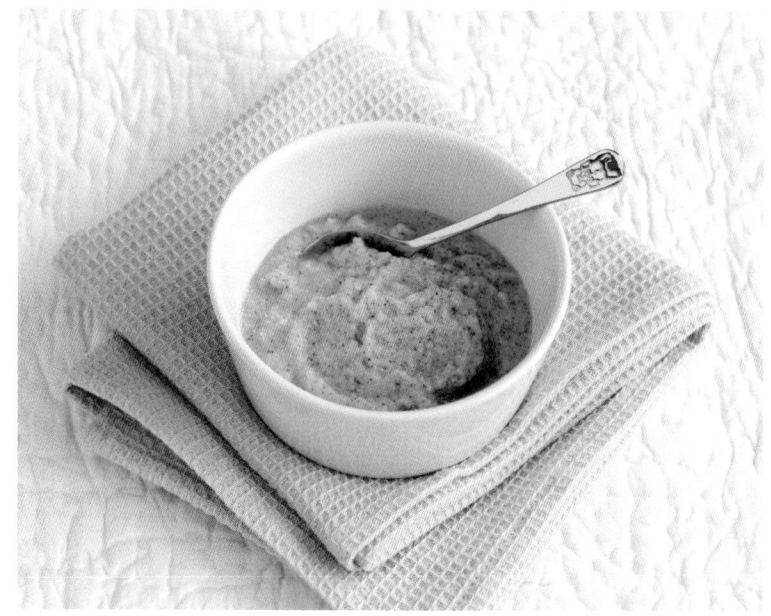

beef, carrot and kumara purée

PREPARATION TIME **10 MINUTES** COOKING TIME **20 MINUTES** MAKES **2 CUPS**

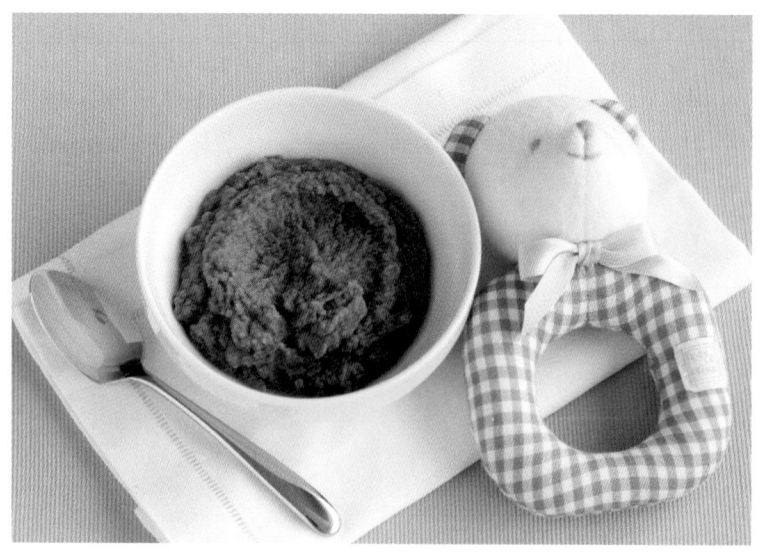

150g beef rump steak, diced
into 3cm pieces

½ small kumara (125g),
chopped coarsely

1 large carrot (180g),
chopped coarsely

1½ cups (375ml) water

1 Place ingredients in small
saucepan; bring to a boil.
Boil, uncovered, until
vegetables soften and
beef is cooked through.

2 Blend or process mixture
until smooth.

fish, potato and spinach purée

PREPARATION TIME **10 MINUTES**
COOKING TIME **20 MINUTES**
MAKES **2 CUPS**

1 large potato (300g),
   chopped coarsely

1½ cups (375ml) water

100g firm white fish fillet,
   chopped coarsely

30g baby spinach leaves

¼ cup (60ml) water, extra

1 Place potato and the water
   in small saucepan; bring to
   a boil. Boil, uncovered, until
   potato is tender; strain potato
   over small bowl.
2 Return liquid to same pan
   with fish and spinach; boil,
   uncovered, until fish is
   cooked through. Drain.
3 Push potato through sieve into
   small bowl. Blend or process
   fish and spinach until smooth;
   stir fish mixture and the extra
   water into potato.

TIPS Freeze any unused purée in
1-tablespoon batches in ice-cube
trays, covered, for up to 1 month.

Make sure any skin and bones
have been removed from the fish
before cooking.

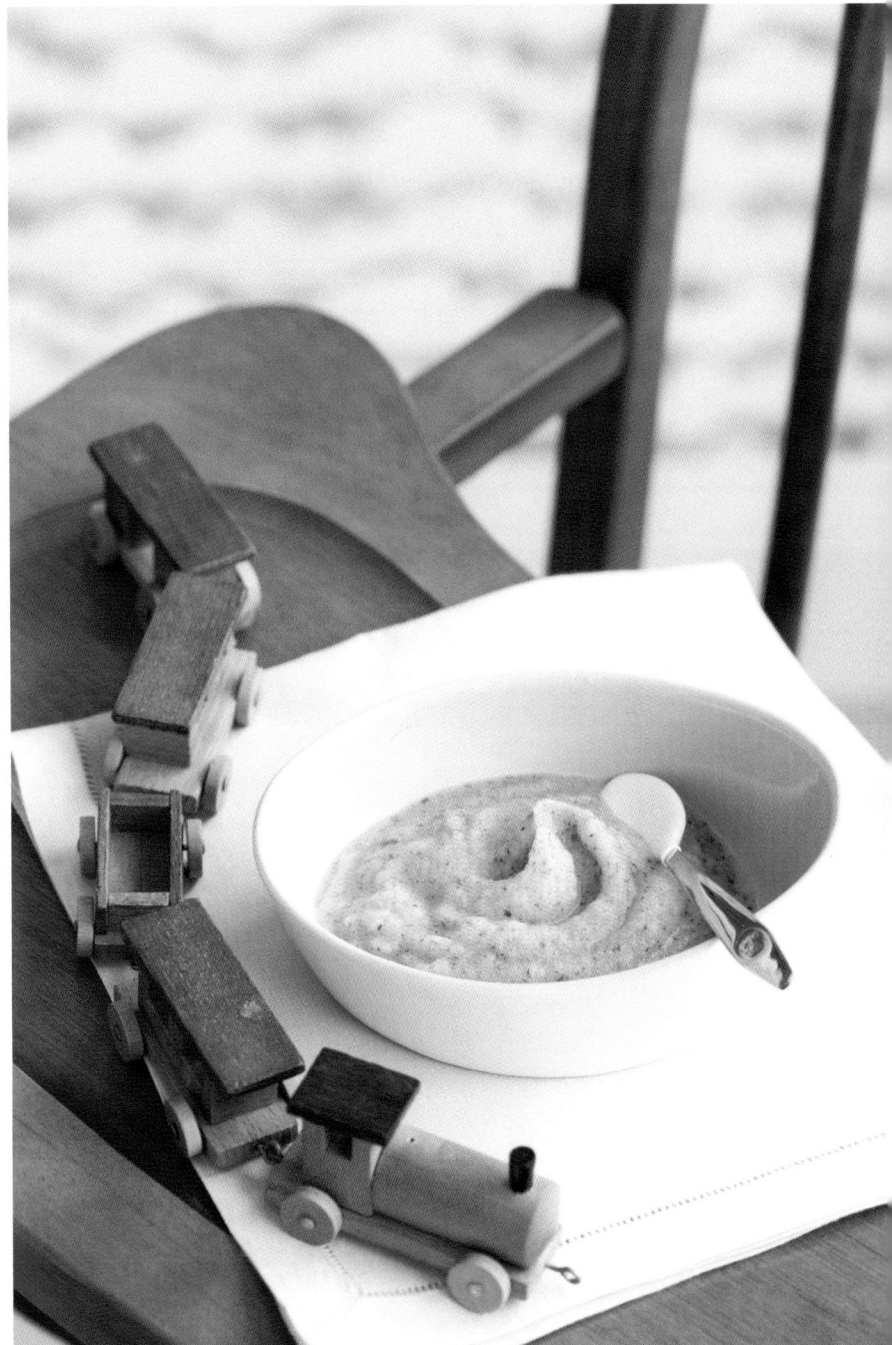

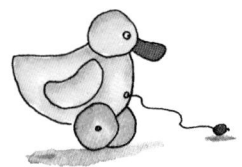

apple with rice cereal

PREPARATION TIME 10 MINUTES (PLUS STANDING TIME) COOKING TIME 10 MINUTES
MAKES ¼ CUP RICE CEREAL; 1 CUP APPLE PUREE

1 tablespoon brown rice flour

1 cup (250ml) water

2 large apples (400g),
    chopped coarsely

1 Blend brown rice flour
   with the water in small
   saucepan; stir over heat until
   mixture boils and thickens.
   Cool to room temperature.
2 Meanwhile, boil, steam
   or microwave apple until
   tender; drain, push through
   sieve into small bowl.
3 Combine 1 tablespoon rice
   cereal with 1 tablespoon
   apple purée to serve.

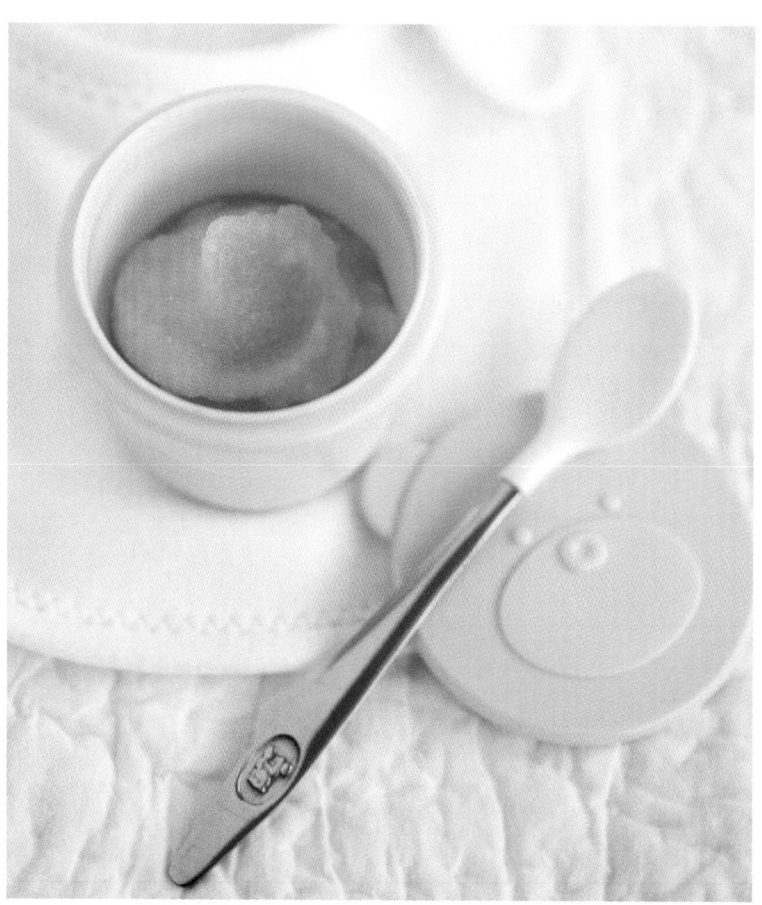

BE LUKEWARM ABOUT IT!

*A microwave oven is a beautiful thing when it comes to defrosting or heating food for
your baby or toddler. But there is an inherent danger in heating food this way (which is
why microwave ovens are not recommended for reheating bottles).*
*Microwaves distribute heat irregularly through food, and the result is that pockets of food
can be super-hot while other pockets can be just lukewarm. After microwaving food, it is very
important to thoroughly stir it to distribute the heat evenly. Then, you should ALWAYS test
the temperature against your skin (dip in a clean finger, or place a small quantity of food
on your lower lip) – it should feel warm, not hot.*

banana with semolina

PREPARATION TIME 10 MINUTES (PLUS STANDING TIME)
COOKING TIME 5 MINUTES
MAKES ⅓ CUP SEMOLINA;
2½ TABLESPOONS BANANA PUREE

2 teaspoons ground semolina
⅓ cup (80ml) water
1 small overripe banana (130g)

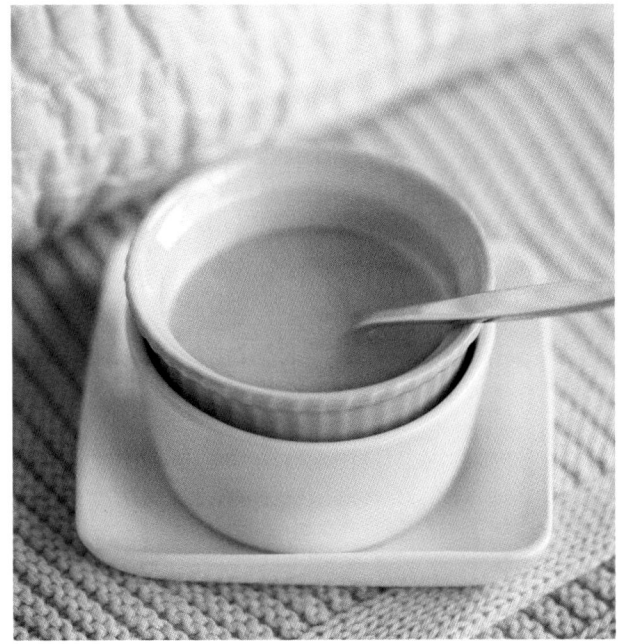

1 Blend semolina and the water in small saucepan; stir over heat until mixture boils and thickens. Cool to room temperature.
2 Push banana through sieve into small bowl.
3 Combine 1 tablespoon semolina with 1 tablespoon banana purée to serve.

egg-yolk custard

PREPARATION TIME 5 MINUTES COOKING TIME 15 MINUTES MAKES ¾ CUP

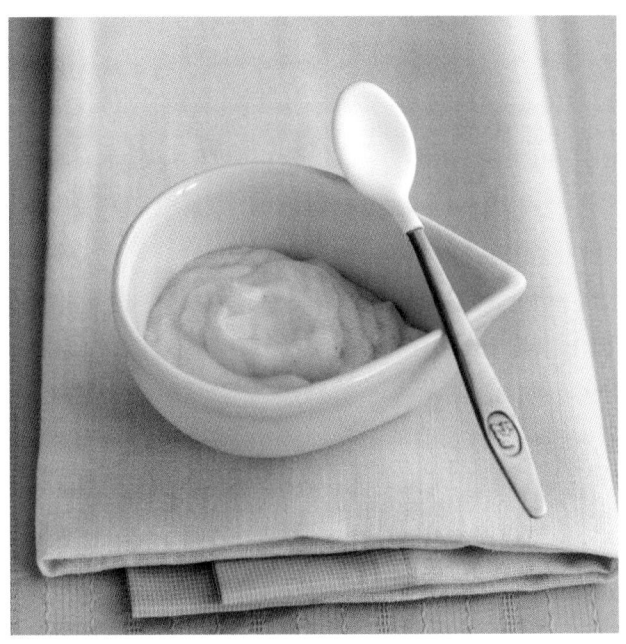

⅔ cup (160ml) milk
pinch ground cinnamon
1 egg yolk
2 teaspoons white sugar
1 teaspoon cornflour

1 Bring milk and cinnamon to a boil in small saucepan; remove from heat.
2 Whisk yolk, sugar and cornflour in small bowl until combined.
3 Pour milk mixture over yolk mixture, whisking continuously until combined.
4 Return mixture to same pan; cook, stirring over low heat, until mixture just boils and thickens. Remove from heat; cover surface of custard with plastic wrap. Cool to room temperature.

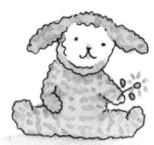

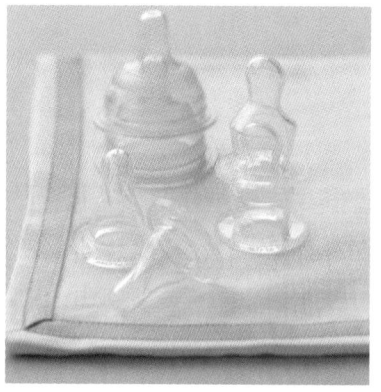
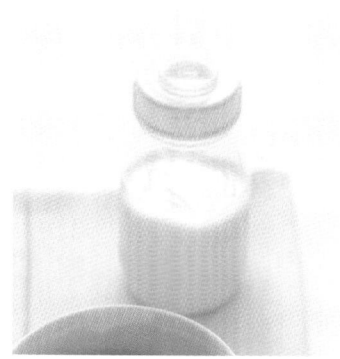
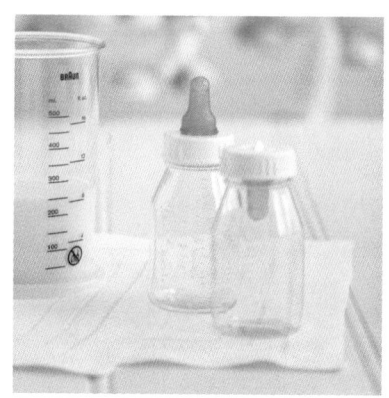

Keep it CLEAN!

Babies are much more vulnerable to germs than adults are – this is why the sterilisation of bottles is highly recommended for the first 12 months. When it comes to general food preparation, following the principles of good hygiene will go a long way towards protecting your baby's good health.

* First and foremost, always wash your hands immediately before preparing food for your child. It sounds obvious, but bacteria can be transferred so easily.

* Make sure that your kitchen utensils are sparkling clean, and be sure to use two chopping boards – one for trimming and chopping raw meats, and the other for the remainder of foods. To clean the boards, always use hot running water and allow to air dry.

* Don't keep leftovers for any longer than 48 hours. Anything left longer is decidedly dodgy and is best thrown out.

* Warm food needs to be cooled as quickly as possible to prevent the spread of bacteria.

The best way to do this is to put the warm food into a shallow container, then straight into the fridge.

* The rear of the refrigerator is the coolest spot, so be sure to always store your child's prepared foods, covered, here. Pay careful attention, also, to the placement of bottles of expressed breastmilk or formula – never leave them in the door of the fridge, as this is the warmest spot.

* When you want to reheat food, make sure you bring it to boiling point, then allow to cool slightly before eating. All food contains some degree of bacterium, most of which are killed by bringing food to boiling point. If using the microwave oven to reheat food, stir it, then allow to stand for a while to make sure there are no "hot spots". Microwaving bottles is not recommended because of this risk of uneven heating.

* When it comes to defrosting, it's a big no-no to leave a packet of mince (or frozen baby food) out at room temperature to thaw. Bacteria love room temperature!

There are two safe ways to defrost: one is to defrost using the microwave, the other is to place the frozen food in the refrigerator to slowly thaw. The latter requires that you plan ahead… you'll need to place the frozen chicken breast for tomorrow night's dinner in the fridge tonight.

* Don't keep pre-made formula for longer than 24 hours. If a bottle has been used for a feed, discard anything that remains after an hour.

* Don't heat bottles or keep bottles warm for longer than 10 minutes. When you go out, take water and infant formula powder separately.

* Don't put any food that has already been heated up back in the fridge for later – dish out only what you need, and throw away any leftovers.

* Make sure that minced meat, poultry and fish is well cooked for young children.

* Honey should not be given to children less than one year of age, because it carries with it a risk of botulism.

Getting out and about

On certain days, going out with a baby or small child can seem all too hard. But if you plan ahead (and cover all contingencies), you can have a pleasant and successful outing to a local cafe or your favourite restaurant.

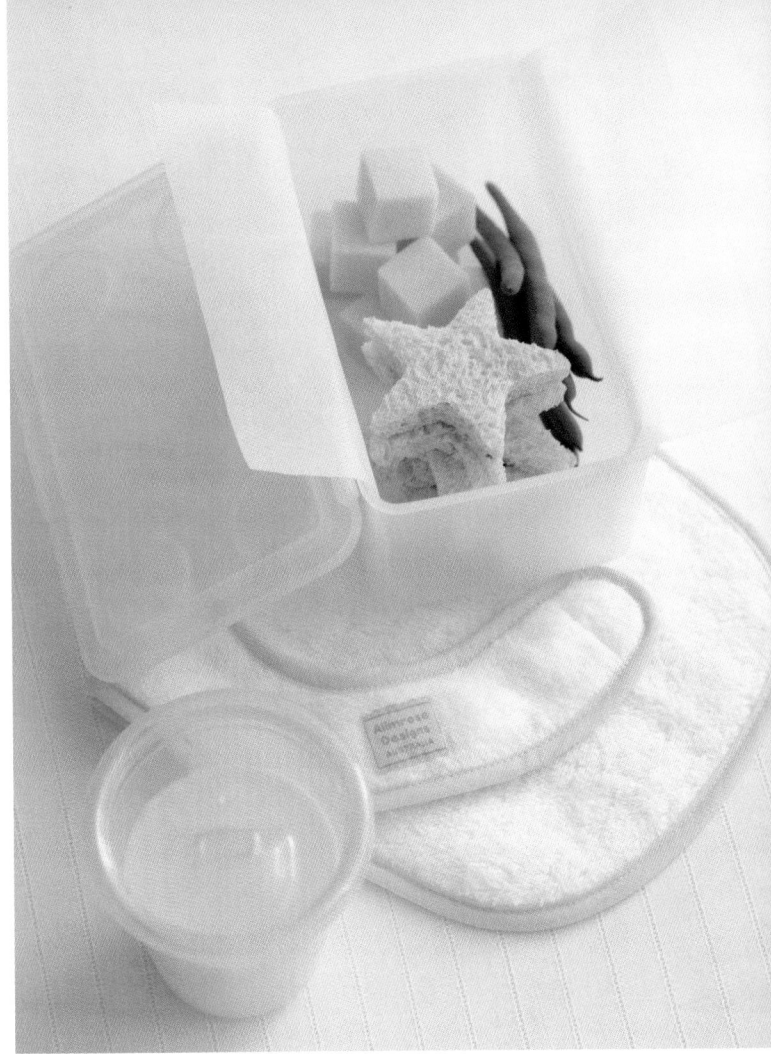

✻ Where possible, change and feed your child just before leaving the house.

✻ If your baby is breastfed, consider whether you will feel comfortable feeding at your destination. If not, pack a bottle of expressed breastmilk with freezer bricks in an insulated cool pack. If bottle-feeding, take water and formula sachets (or a pre-measured quantity of powder) to mix as and when you need it – there is a greater risk of bacteria breeding in ready-mixed formula. To give your baby a warm feed, ask the staff to provide a small amount of boiled water to add to the water in the bottle, or to warm the bottle for you.

✻ If your baby has moved onto solid foods, pack a range of snacks. For the six-month-plus age group (often still toothless), pack plain dried biscuits (try breadsticks or arrowroots) and homemade rusks – you'll be delighted by how long it can take a toothless child to suck a biscuit into submission! Supplement with either a drink of water or milk (formula or breast). If your baby's need for a full meal coincides with your outing, take along a spoon and a jar of commercial baby food (such convenience will work wonders for your stress levels) or pack up some homemade food that can be kept chilled until it is required.

✻ Once your child has hit toddlerhood, take along some of their favourite foods. Cheese, vegemite sandwiches, rice cakes, steamed vegetables… Focus on finger foods that they can manage themselves – it will make your visit far easier. They may end up messy but, as a parent, you'll invariably carry wipes to clean up messy faces and hands. For a drink, most toddlers will feel terribly grown-up while sipping on a milkshake (request a half-serving and pour it into a cup brought from home). Alternatively, pack a "popper" of milk or juice, and you'll be laughing as you sip your latte.

✻ Remember that restaurants and cafes are in the business of customer service so, if you ask nicely, most restaurants will be only too happy to reheat your baby's meal in their microwave. A word of warning on this, though… commercial microwave ovens (found in most cafes and restaurants) are far more powerful than most microwave ovens in the home, so be terribly conservative with the time that you request the food/drink be heated for, and stir it thoroughly and then test the temperature on your skin before feeding it to your child.

✻ One other tip to make your outing a success is to give the restaurant/cafe some notice that you intend on bringing a stroller or pram to their premises. They may need to rearrange tables to fit you in and, if they can organise this prior to your arrival, there will be no need to disturb their other patrons. It's a simple courtesy that benefits everybody.

Now, go out and have fun!

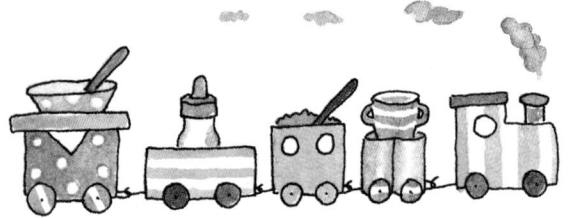

8-12 MONTHS

Now that your baby is eating solid foods, it's time to raise the stakes and start experimenting with texture and flavour. The recipes in this chapter demonstrate how easy it is to gradually and safely introduce foods that encourage a keen appetite and enthusiastic chewing.

Texture

Once your baby is happily consuming a range of different foods, it's time to experiment with texture. Try feeding your baby cooked vegetables that have been only roughly mashed with a fork, so the soft lumps will encourage them to chew their food. Initially, you may find your baby gags and brings the food back up – this is a reflex that he will quickly overcome through your persistence. And no, it won't matter if your child is yet to teethe – babies can chew quite efficiently using only their gums.

Once small lumps have been mastered, try offering your baby small pieces of steamed vegetables, soft fruit, bread or meat, as finger food.

Drinking from cups

There is no requirement that you teach your baby to drink from a cup by a certain age, but there are some undeniable advantages to achieving this in the first year (such as being able to get rid of bottles).

A cup is any drinking receptacle that does not have a teat – so a small cup, or a container with a spout or a straw.

Start by offering your baby just a couple of teaspoons of liquid in a small cup – you'll need to hold the cup to their lips and tip it up. A common reaction from babies is that they'll happily take the liquid into their mouth, but it will then dribble straight back out. Babies need to learn to close their mouth and swallow, so your gentle persistence will pay off. Don't expect your child to go even close to drinking the quantity that they have been taking from a bottle or breastfeed – this will take time. The aim is just to teach your baby what to do, not to replace all feeds immediately with cup drinking. The more patience you can exercise and the more frequently your baby has the opportunity to practice, the faster he will get the hang of it.

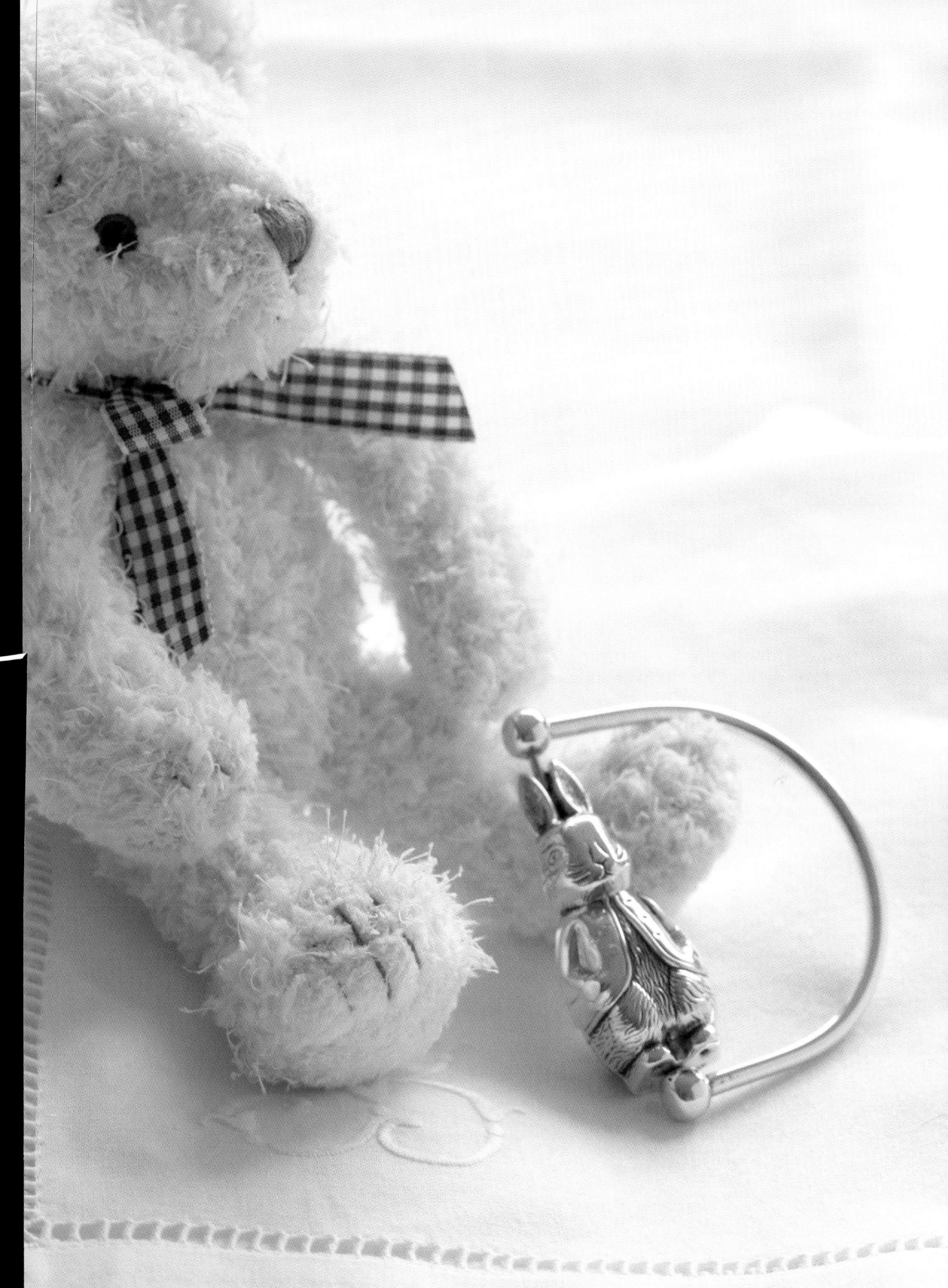

PUREES MADE EASY

The tables on these two pages have been created so you can quickly and easily make your purée of choice, according to the groupings of fruit or vegetable. Read down the first column on the left of each table to find your ingredient of choice, then read across to discover the quantity you'll need, the preparation technique and the time it will take to cook. For a purée that could be slightly gluggy, we've also suggested what quantity of liquid you'll need to add to make it easier for your baby to manage.

fruit purées

ALL PUREES MAKE 1 CUP
(12 TABLESPOONS)

For apple and pear:

1 Combine fruit and the water in medium saucepan; bring to a boil. Reduce heat; simmer, uncovered, until tender.
2 Blend or process fruit mixture until smooth. Give your child as much fruit purée as desired.

For remaining fruit:

Blend or process fruit until smooth. Give your child as much fruit purée as desired.

TIP Fruit and vegetable purées can be frozen in 1-tablespoon batches in ice-cube trays, covered, for up to 1 month.

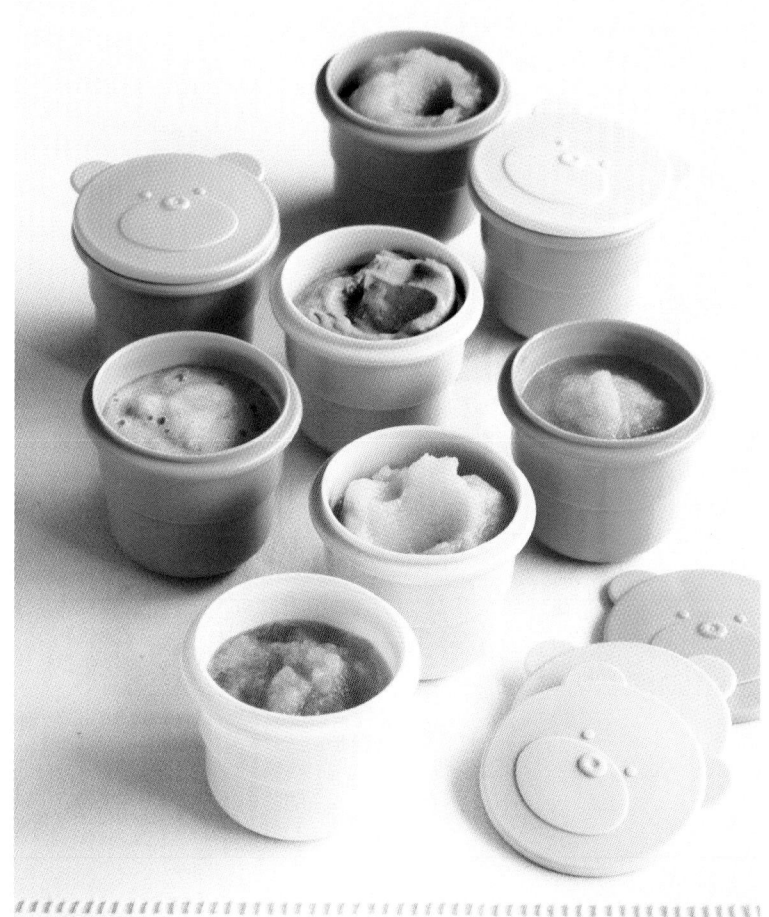

FRUIT	QUANTITY	PREPARATION	COOKING TIME	WATER
Apple	2 large (400g)	Peel, core, chop coarsely	10 minutes	2 tablespoons
Avocado	2 small (400g)	Peel, seed, chop coarsely	-	-
Banana	2 medium (400g)	Peel, chop coarsely	-	-
Custard apple	400g	Peel, seed, chop coarsely	-	-
Pear	1 large (330g)	Peel, core, chop coarsely	20 minutes	2 tablespoons
Rockmelon	500g	Peel (remove all green sections), seed, chop coarsely	-	-

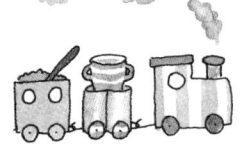

fruit mash

ALL MASH RECIPES MAKE 1 CUP (12 TABLESPOONS)

For apple and prune:
1 Combine apple, prune and the water in medium saucepan; bring to a boil. Reduce heat; simmer, covered, until apple and prune are tender.
2 Blend, process or mash apple mixture until desired consistency. Give your child as much fruit mash as desired.

For blueberry:
1 Combine blueberries and the water in medium saucepan; bring to a boil. Reduce heat; simmer, uncovered, until softened.
2 Push blueberries through sieve in small bowl. Give your child as much fruit mash as desired.

For strawberry:
1 Combine strawberries and juice in medium saucepan; bring to a boil. Reduce heat; simmer, uncovered, until softened.
2 Push strawberries through sieve in small bowl. Give your child as much fruit mash as desired.

For remaining fruits:
1 Blend, process or mash fruit (and liquid) until desired consistency. Give your child as much fruit mash as desired.

TIP Freeze any unused mash in 1-tablespoon batches in ice-cube trays, covered, for up to 1 month.

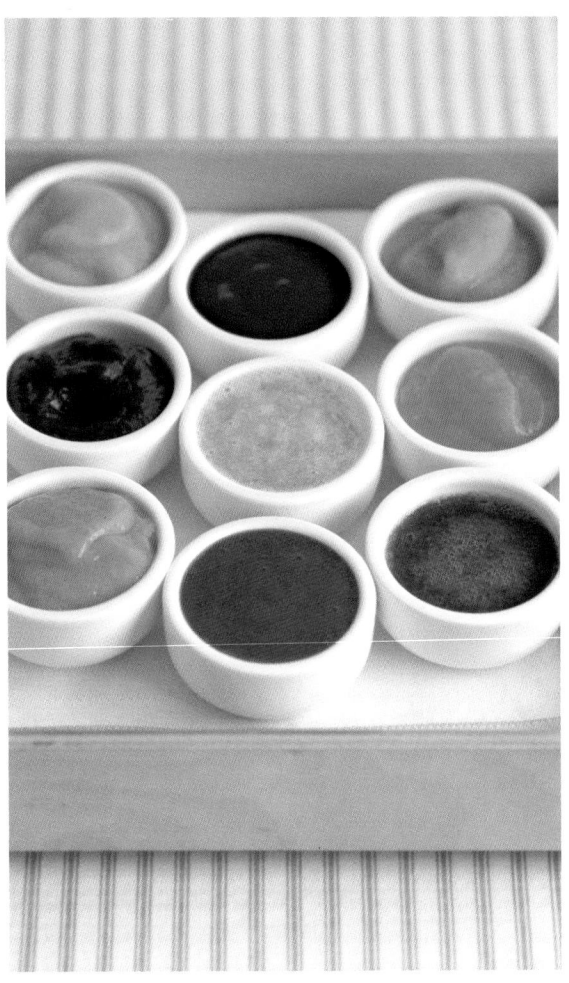

FRUIT	QUANTITY	PREPARATION	COOKING TIME	LIQUID
Apple and prune	2 large apples (400g) ⅓ cup (55g) seeded prunes	Apple: peel, core, slice thinly Prunes: chop coarsely	15 minutes	¼ cup water
Apricot	425g can, drained	-	-	-
Blueberry	300g	Chop coarsely	5 minutes	2 tablespoons water
Grape (seedless)	250g	Chop coarsely	-	-
Mandarin	2 medium (400g)	Peel, discard pith, seed	-	1 tablespoon apple juice
Mango	2 small (600g)	Peel, seed, chop coarsely	-	-
Papaya	1 small (650g)	Peel, seed, chop coarsely	-	-
Peach	425g can, drained	-	-	-
Strawberry	375g	Chop coarsely	5 minutes	¼ cup apple juice

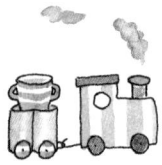

mash combinations

ALL COMBINATIONS MAKE ⅓ CUP (4 TABLESPOONS)

All of the mash combinations on these pages
are made using the completed fruit and vegetable
mashes that feature on the previous pages (32-33).

vegetable and cheese

Combine 1 tablespoon mashed asparagus,
1 tablespoon mashed parsnip and 1 tablespoon
mashed pea; top with 1 tablespoon finely
grated tasty cheese.

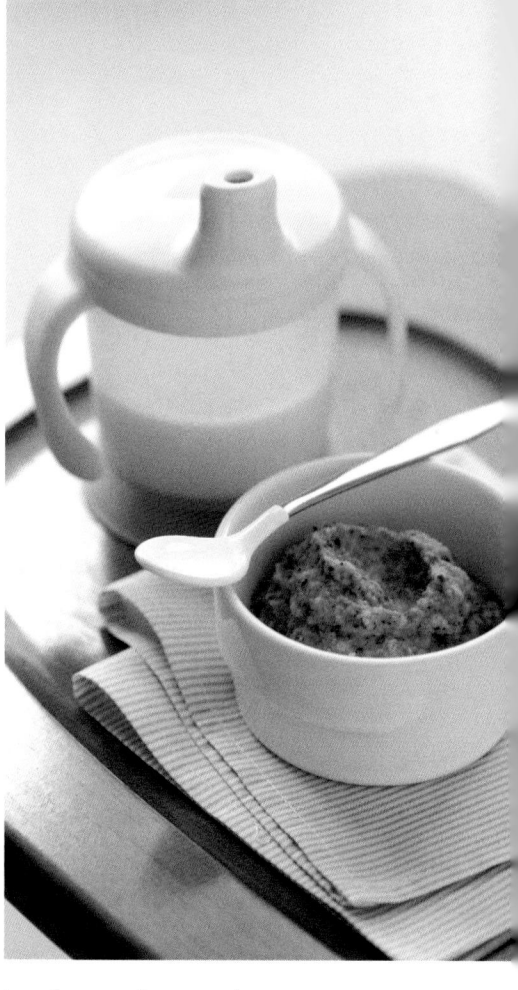

leek and mushroom

Combine 3 tablespoons mashed leek with
1 tablespoon mashed mushroom.

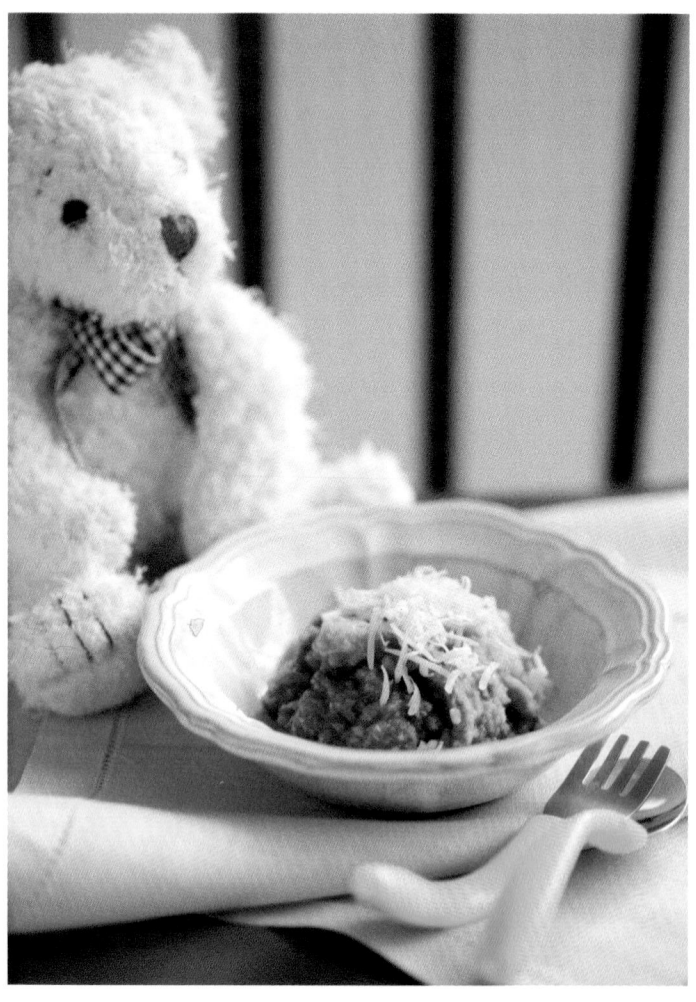

fruit yogurt

Combine 1 tablespoon mashed strawberry, 1 tablespoon mashed blueberry and 2 tablespoons natural or vanilla yogurt.

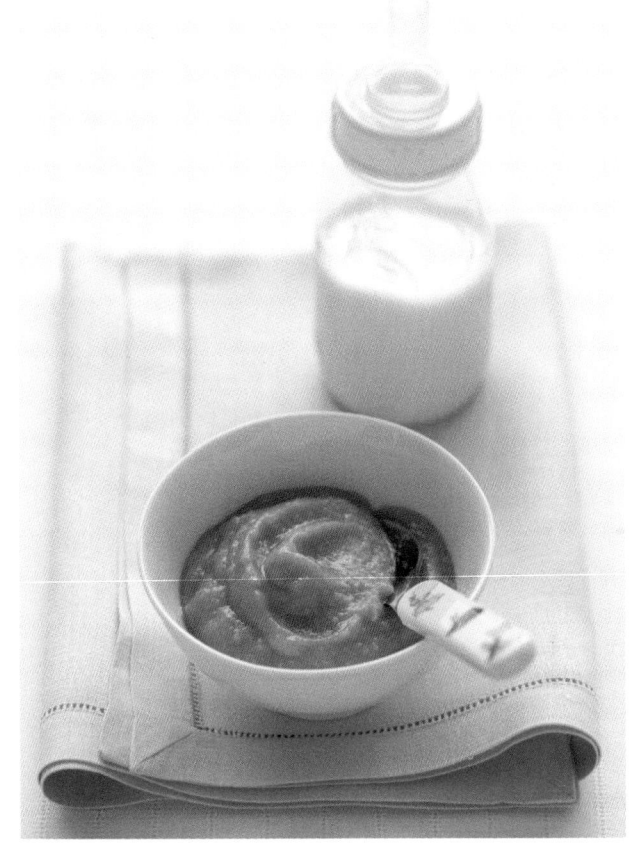

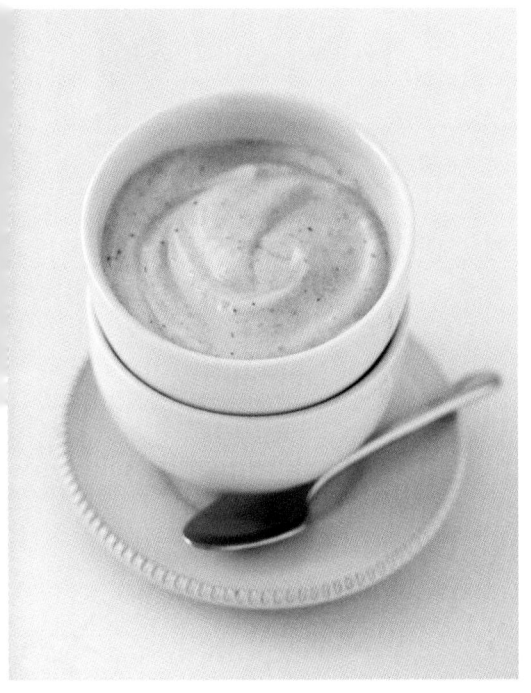

pumpkin and sweet corn

Combine 2 tablespoons mashed canned creamed corn with 2 tablespoons puréed pumpkin (see page 21).

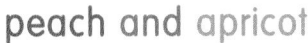

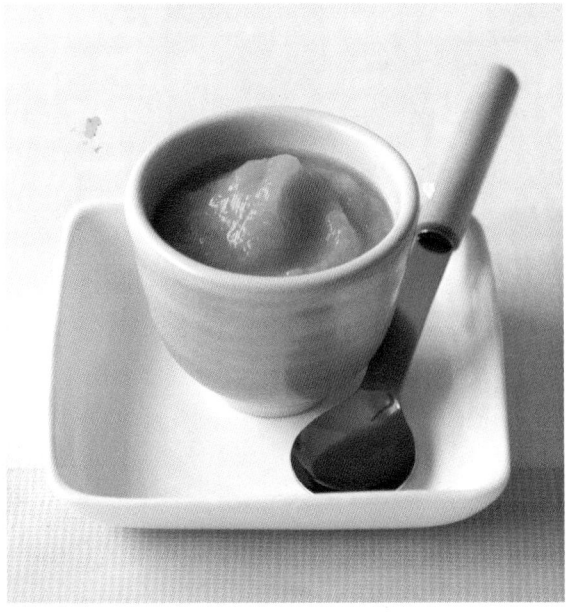

peach and apricot

Combine 2 tablespoons mashed apricot with 2 tablespoons mashed peach.

Safety first

Food is a wonderful, sharing part of life, but it does present a few hazards to your baby or toddler. Aside from the threat of food allergies (read more on page 8), choking is an ongoing danger to your child. Babies and young toddlers are just learning to use their teeth and to properly chew a mouthful prior to swallowing, and their enthusiasm for what they're eating can often lead to an attempt to swallow things whole, or to inhale food or drink into the lungs.

Read on for some tips on preventing choking…

✳ Closely supervise your child at all mealtimes, and make sure they sit quietly to eat.

✳ Raw or semi-cooked fruit and vegetables that are particularly hard should be avoided (apple, carrot or celery, for instance). Steam these foods to soften them, or grate them, before offering them to your child.

✳ Don't feed your baby pieces of cheese or meat until they are ready to chew them. Instead, grate or melt cheese through meals, and blend, purée or finely chop meat (this includes mince).

✳ It's time consuming but definitely safer to remove all skin, seeds and pips from fruit. Similarly, remove all bones and skin from meat and fish before giving to your child.

✳ Avoid obvious choking hazards such as whole nuts and peas, popcorn, corn chips, chewing gum, lollies (particularly boiled lollies), whole grapes and large chunks of sausage or frankfurt.

Of course, in the case of babies (who seem to put everything in their mouths), choking isn't related solely to food consumption. You should take great care to put away all small objects that may tempt your baby, for example, buttons, coins, pins, beads and a wide variety of other objects.

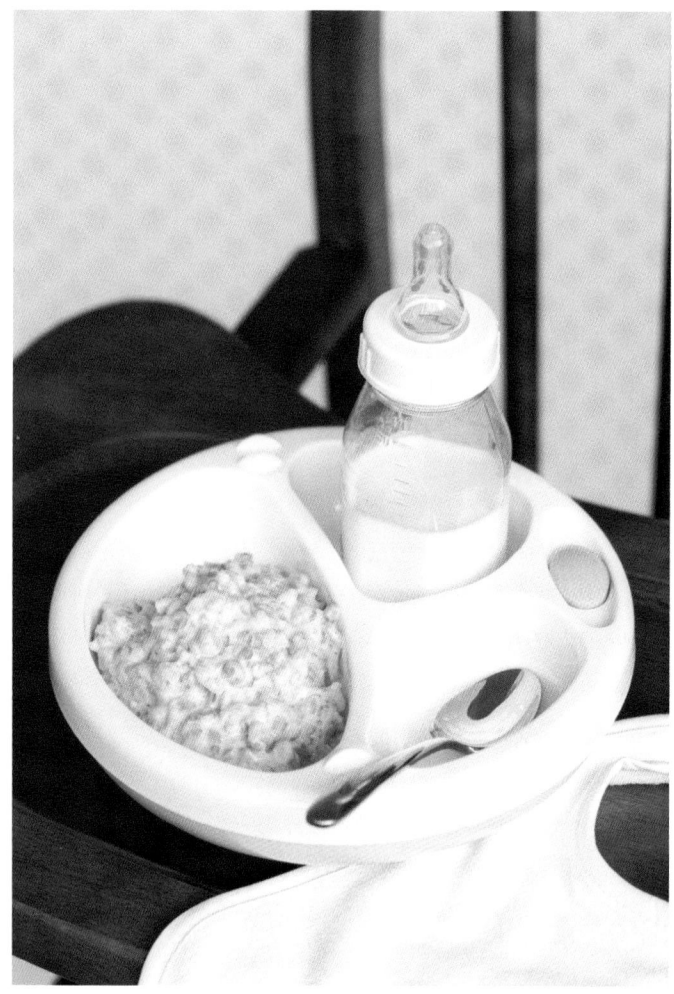

oat porridge

PREPARATION TIME 5 MINUTES   COOKING TIME 10 MINUTES   MAKES ½ CUP

⅓ cup (80g) rolled oats
¾ cup (180ml) milk

1 Combine ingredients in small saucepan; bring to a boil.
2 Reduce heat; simmer, uncovered, about 8 minutes or until all liquid is almost absorbed. Cool.

TIP Add a little cold milk just before serving if porridge is too thick.

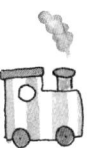

risoni with mixed vegetables

PREPARATION TIME 10 MINUTES COOKING TIME 20 MINUTES
MAKES ⅓ CUP RISONI 1½ CUPS VEGETABLE MIXTURE

1 small red capsicum (150g), chopped finely

1 large zucchini (150g), chopped finely

310g can corn kernels, drained

400g can crushed tomatoes

2 tablespoons risoni

1 Cook capsicum in medium heated lightly oiled non-stick frying pan, stirring, 3 minutes. Add zucchini and corn; cook, stirring, 2 minutes. Add undrained tomatoes; cook, stirring occasionally, about 15 minutes or until vegetables soften. Blend or process until smooth.

2 Meanwhile, cook risoni in small saucepan of boiling water, uncovered, until tender; drain.

3 Toss risoni with ¼ cup of the vegetable mixture.

TIP Freeze the vegetable mixture in ¼-cup batches, covered, for up to 1 month.

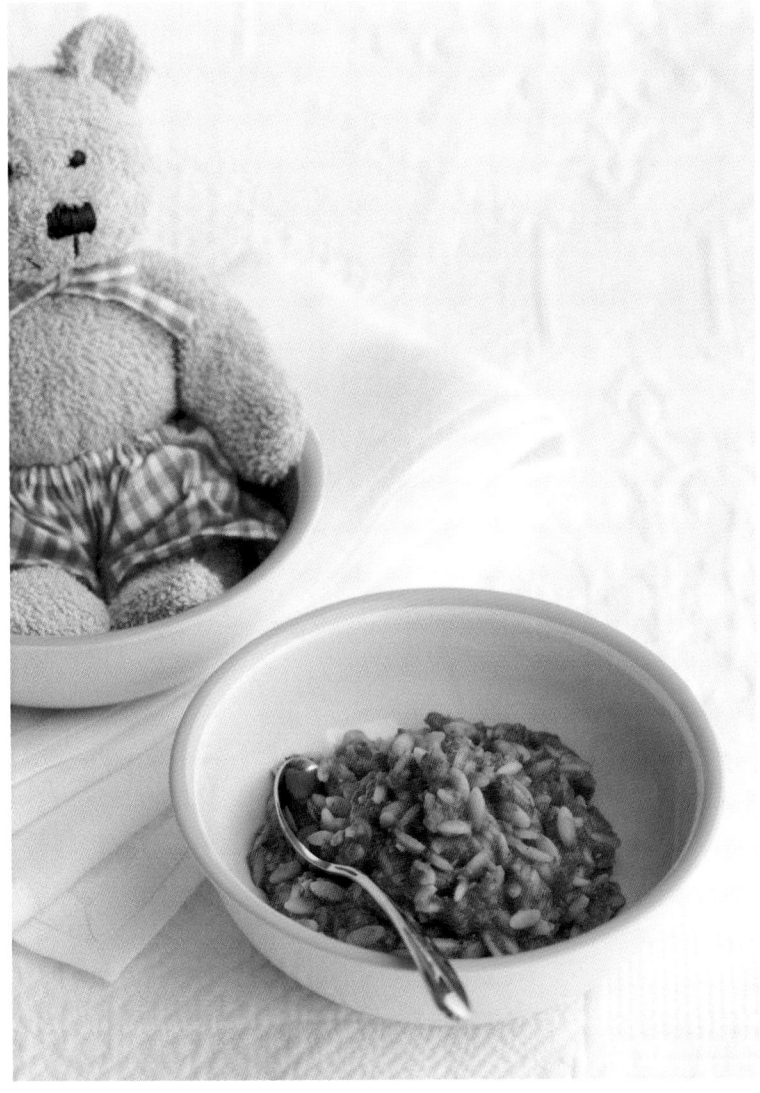

creamy cheese polenta

PREPARATION TIME 5 MINUTES
(PLUS STANDING TIME)
COOKING TIME 15 MINUTES
MAKES 1 CUP

1 cup (250ml) water
1½ cups (375ml) milk
⅓ cup (55g) polenta
¼ cup (30g) coarsely
   grated cheddar

1 Combine the water and milk in small saucepan; bring to a boil. Gradually add polenta to liquid, stirring constantly.
2 Reduce heat; simmer, stirring, about 10 minutes or until polenta thickens. Stir in cheese, cover; cool 10 minutes, stirring occasionally.

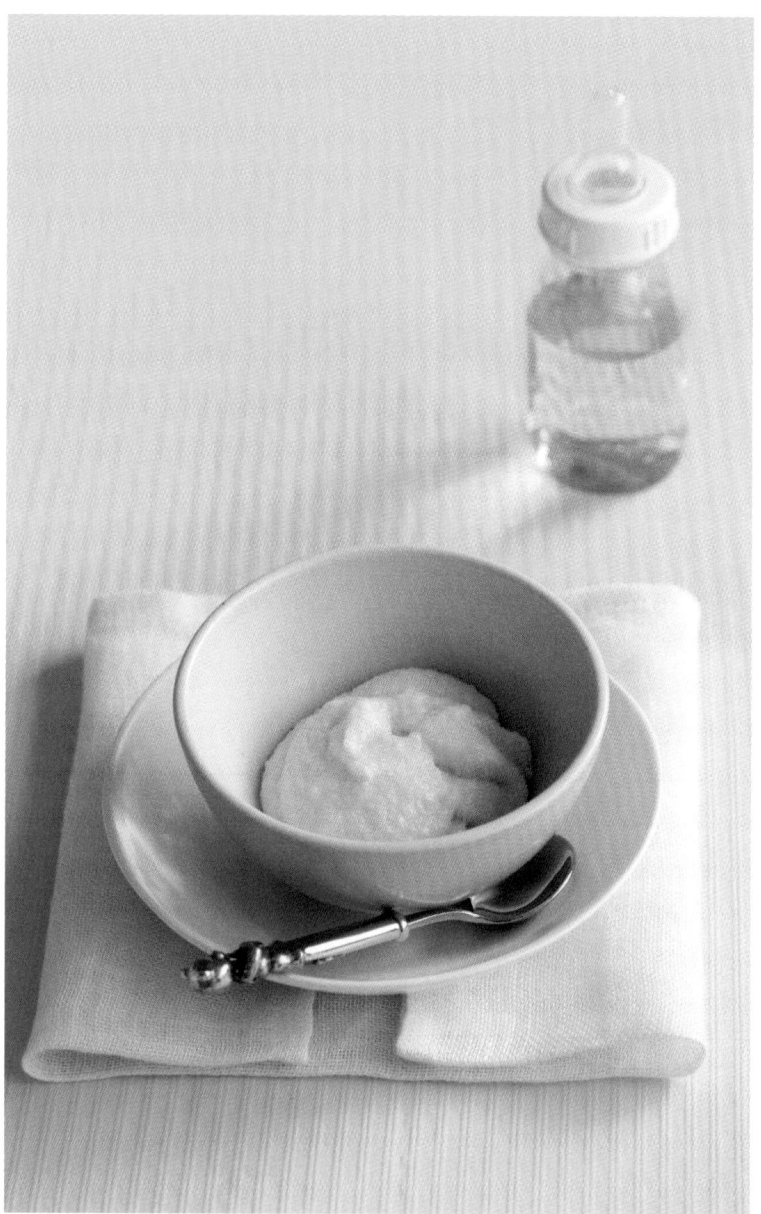

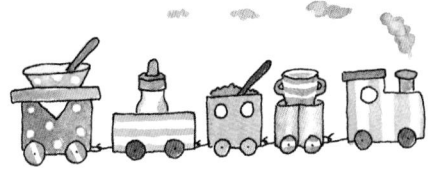

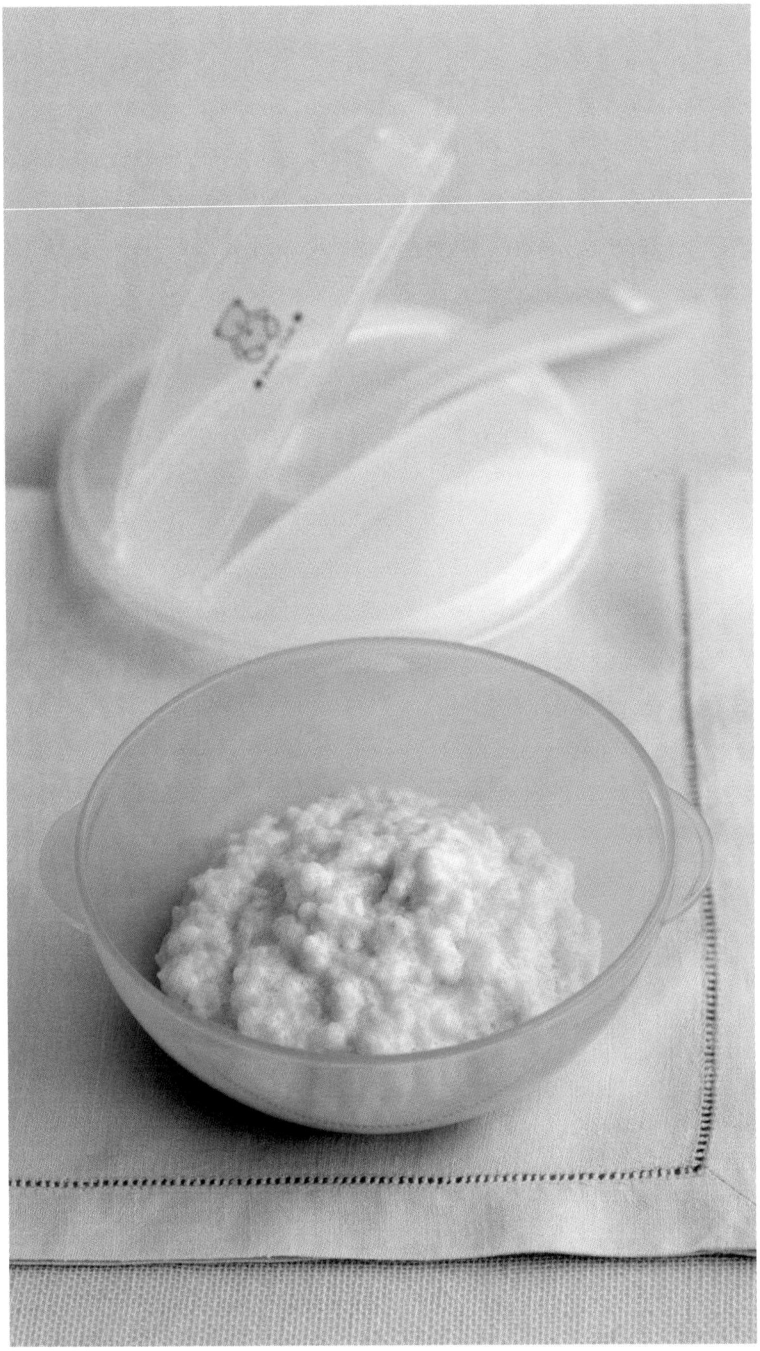

sweet
COUSCOUS

PREPARATION TIME 10 MINUTES
COOKING TIME 10 MINUTES
MAKES ⅓ CUP

1 cup (250ml) milk
1 tablespoon couscous
1 teaspoon white sugar
pinch ground cinnamon

1 Combine ingredients in small
   saucepan; bring to a boil.
2 Reduce heat; simmer, stirring,
   about 10 minutes or until
   mixture thickens.

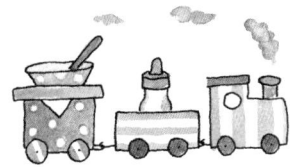

scrambled egg

PREPARATION TIME 3 MINUTES   COOKING TIME 3 MINUTES   MAKES ⅓ CUP

1 egg
2 tablespoons milk
5g butter

1 Combine egg and milk in small bowl.
2 Heat butter in small frying pan; cook egg mixture, stirring, over low heat, until egg sets.

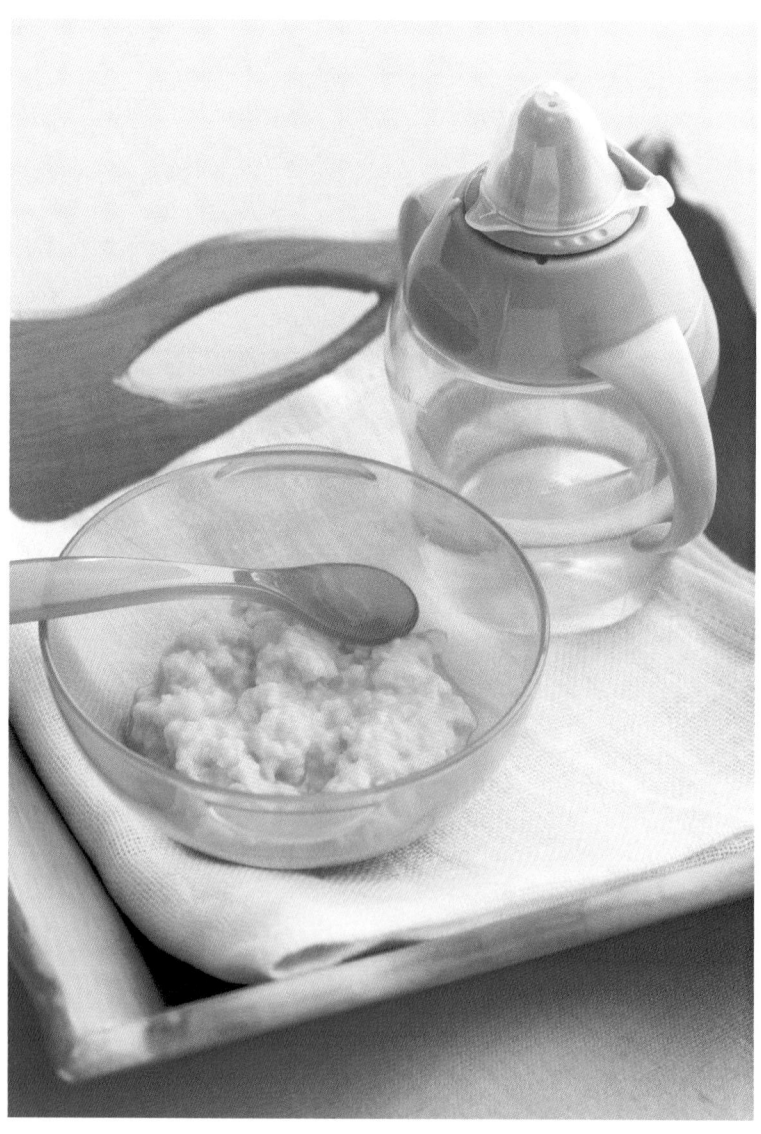

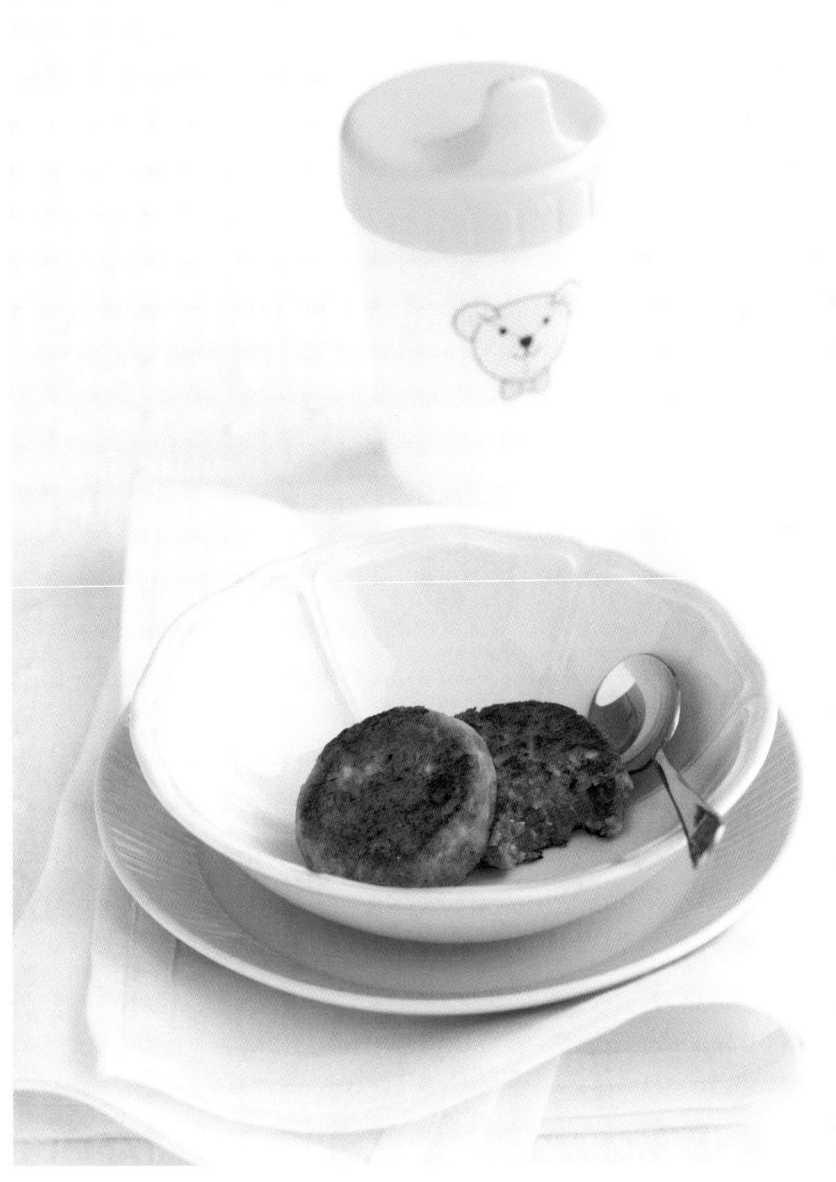

tofu and vegetable patties

PREPARATION TIME 10 MINUTES COOKING TIME 10 MINUTES MAKES 2

1 tablespoon mashed silken tofu

1 tablespoon mashed kumara

1 tablespoon mashed carrot

1 tablespoon puréed zucchini

2 teaspoons rice flour

1 Combine ingredients in small bowl; shape into two patties.

2 Heat small lightly oiled non-stick frying pan; cook patties, uncovered, about 3 minutes each side or until heated through and browned lightly.

TIP Use any vegetables that you may already have, just be sure to use a total of ¼ cup (3 tablespoons) cooked mashed vegetables.

baked ricotta with tomato sauce

PREPARATION TIME 10 MINUTES COOKING TIME 20 MINUTES MAKES 4

400g ricotta

1 tablespoon finely chopped
   fresh oregano

1 tablespoon olive oil

1 clove garlic, crushed

425g can diced tomatoes

½ cup (130g) bottled tomato
   pasta sauce

1 teaspoon white sugar

1 Preheat oven to moderately
   slow. Line oven tray with
   baking paper.
2 Using hand, combine cheese
   and oregano in small bowl;
   shape mixture into four
   patties. Place on prepared
   tray; drizzle with half of
   the oil. Bake, uncovered,
   in moderately slow oven
   about 20 minutes or until
   heated through.
3 Meanwhile, heat remaining
   oil in small saucepan; cook
   garlic, stirring, 1 minute.
   Add undrained tomatoes,
   pasta sauce and sugar;
   bring to a boil. Reduce
   heat; simmer, uncovered,
   stirring occasionally, about
   15 minutes or until sauce
   thickens. Serve sauce with
   baked ricotta.

TIP Leftover baked ricotta can
be used in pasta, a frittata or
on pizza.

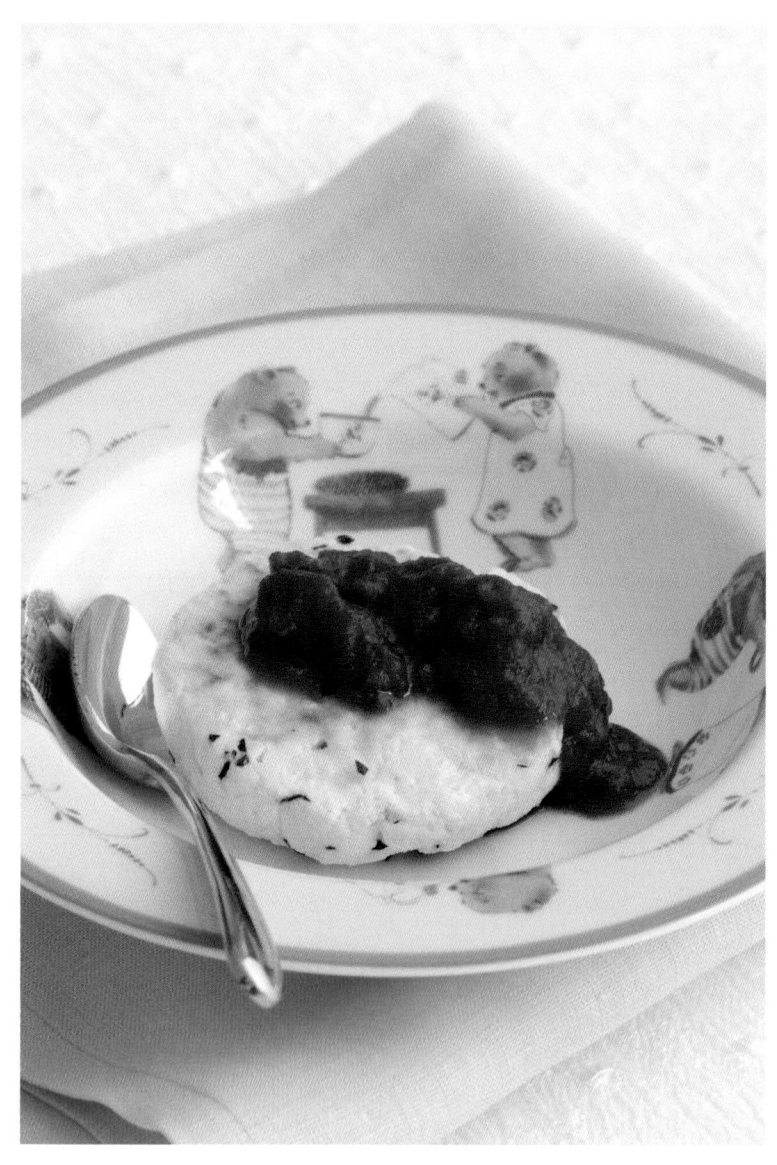

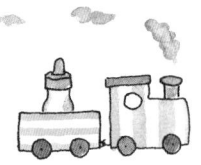

chicken livers with pumpkin

PREPARATION TIME 10 MINUTES (PLUS STANDING TIME)
COOKING TIME 15 MINUTES MAKES 2 CUPS

200g chicken livers
½ cup (125ml) milk
500g pumpkin, chopped coarsely
1 tablespoon olive oil

1 Soak livers in milk in small bowl 30 minutes; drain, discard milk. Separate livers into halves by cutting lobes apart.
2 Meanwhile, boil, steam or microwave pumpkin until just tender; drain.
3 Heat oil in medium frying pan; cook livers, over high heat, about 5 minutes or until cooked through. Drain on absorbent paper.
4 Blend or process pumpkin and livers until smooth, or mash with a fork.

TIP If mixture is too thick, add a little water to obtain desired consistency.

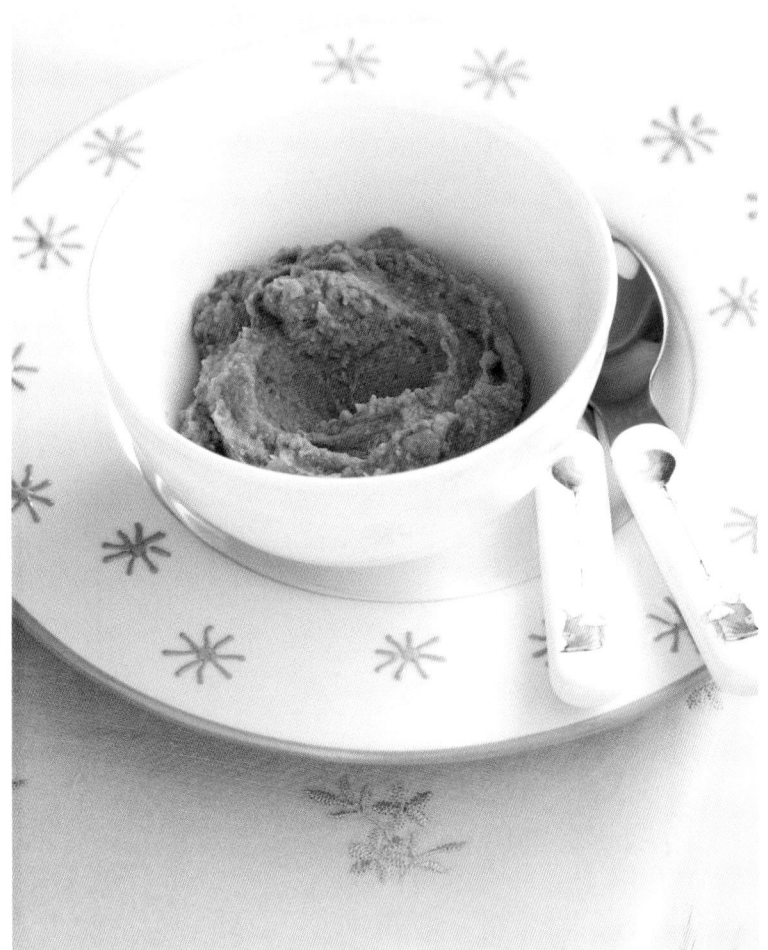

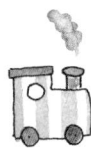

fish in cheese sauce

PREPARATION TIME 5 MINUTES   COOKING TIME 10 MINUTES   MAKES 1 CUP CHEESE SAUCE

10g butter

2 teaspoons plain flour

½ cup (125ml) milk

2 tablespoons finely
  grated cheddar

30g flathead fillet

1 tablespoon small broccoli florets

1 Melt butter in small saucepan, add flour; cook, stirring, until mixture bubbles and thickens. Gradually add milk; cook, stirring, until sauce boils and thickens slightly. Remove from heat; stir in cheese.

2 Meanwhile, boil, steam or microwave fish and broccoli, separately, until broccoli is tender and fish is cooked through; drain.

3 Flake fish into small chunks, carefully removing any bones; combine fish, broccoli and 1 tablespoon of the cheese sauce in small bowl.

TIPS Cheese sauce can also be used on mashed vegetables, puréed chicken or pasta.

Freeze remaining cheese sauce in 1-tablespoon batches in ice-cube trays, covered, for up to 1 month.

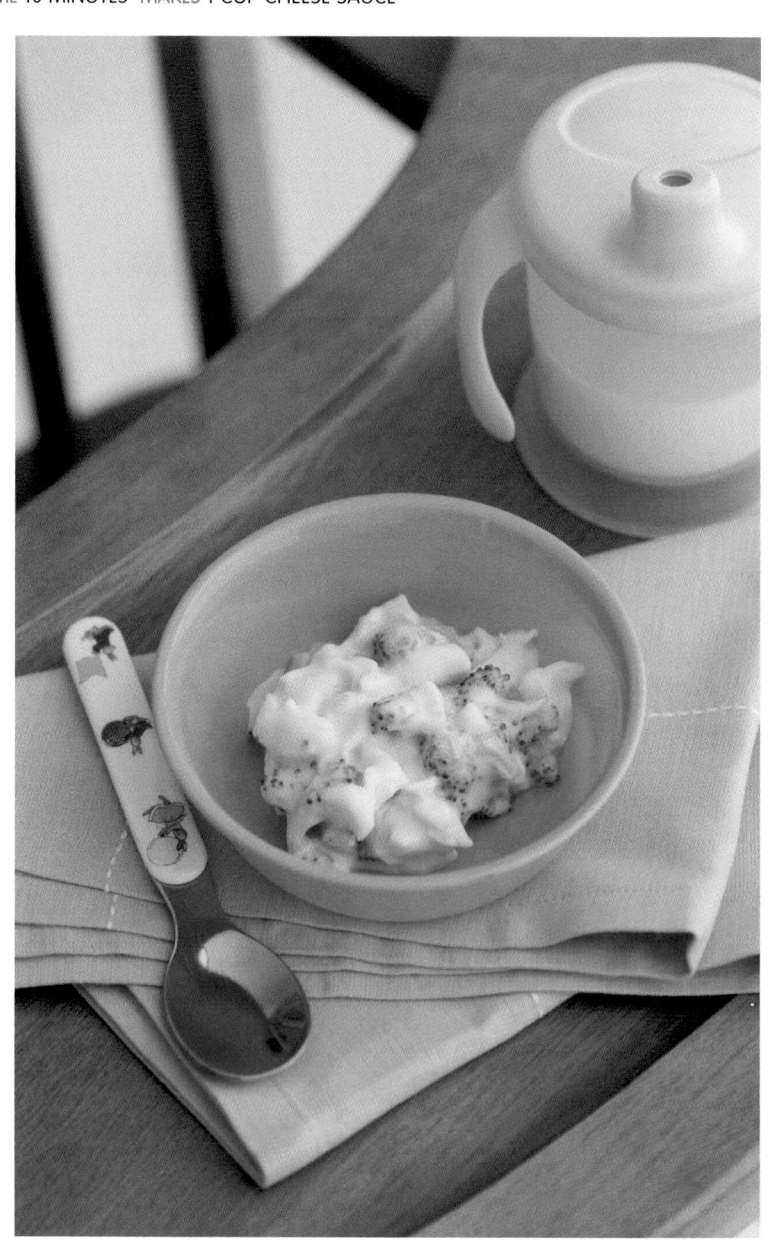

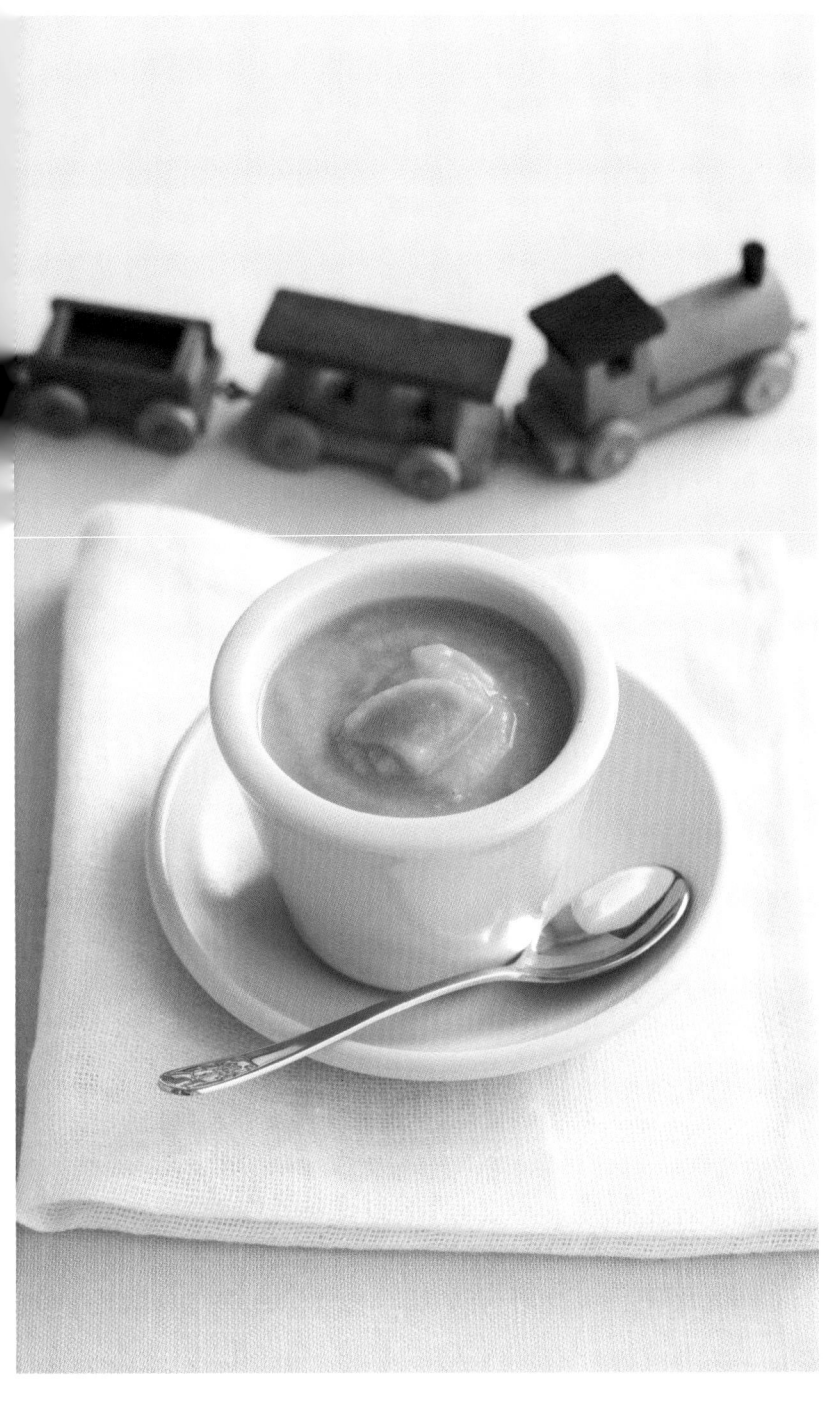

pumpkin and kumara soup

PREPARATION TIME 20 MINUTES
COOKING TIME 25 MINUTES
MAKES 2 CUPS

1 tablespoon olive oil

1 small brown onion (80g), chopped coarsely

1 clove garlic, chopped coarsely

200g pumpkin, chopped coarsely

1 small kumara (250g), chopped coarsely

½ cup (125ml) salt-reduced chicken stock

½ cup (125ml) milk

½ cup (125ml) water

1 Heat oil in small saucepan; cook onion and garlic, stirring, until onion softens. Add pumpkin, kumara and stock; cook, covered, over medium heat, about 15 minutes or until pumpkin and kumara are tender.

2 Blend or process pumpkin mixture until smooth. Return to pan with milk and the water; bring to a boil. Reduce heat; simmer, uncovered, about 5 minutes or until soup is heated through.

TIP Freeze remaining soup in 1-tablespoon batches in ice-cube trays, covered, for up to 2 months.

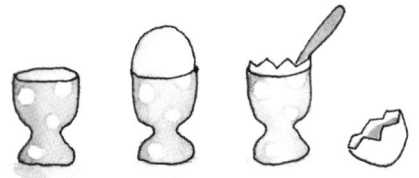

12-24 MONTHS

The good, simple food featured in this chapter is not only easily prepared, it also holds high appeal to young toddlers.

Fussy eaters

If your child is less than keen when it comes to mealtimes, try to take solace in the knowledge that healthy babies and toddlers have the perfect measure of their own appetite; that is, when they're hungry, they'll eat, and when they're thirsty, they'll drink.

That said, parents can still find it terribly worrying when they think their child isn't eating the quantities they should. Food is an emotional topic – we all want our kids to be healthy and active and, quite often, we spend a lot of time preparing nutritious meals to achieve this end. But the fact remains that you can't force a child to eat.

Children can become "fussy" eaters as early as nine months of age and, unfortunately, such a stage is common right through until three years of age, and beyond. So, parents, read through the following tips to make mealtimes just that little bit easier.

- Use appropriate feeding equipment: fork, spoon, plate, cup, highchair and bib.
- Try to keep meals and snacks to regular times each day.
- Ensure that your baby or toddler gets plenty of fresh air and exercise, as well as adequate sleep – these elements all lead to a healthy appetite.
- Does your child reject every new food offered to them? Studies have found that, if you keep offering the food (10 times or more), your child will become familiar with that food, leading to its eventual acceptance into their diet. Do not interpret one rejection of a new food as your child not liking it. Introduce only one new food at a time, and take it slowly.
- Accept that food refusal, especially in toddlers, often comes back to their desire to be willful. A child quickly learns that they can trigger a parental reaction by refusing food.
- Avoid making mealtimes a battle. Family meals should be about sharing and conviviality; if your toddler won't eat, remove his food and excuse him from the table. Your child's fussy ways will not change if they associate mealtimes with anger and disharmony.
- Don't bribe your child to eat their dinner on the promise of dessert.
- Set a good example by serving and eating all manner of foods, regardless of your tastes. If you are seen to reject certain foods, you are giving your child permission to do likewise.

If you are still worried about your child's intake, keep a food diary over the course of a week – write down everything that passes your child's lips. Then visit your local Early Childhood Centre or GP to discuss your concerns; your health professional will measure and weigh your child and, if necessary, offer some helpful advice.

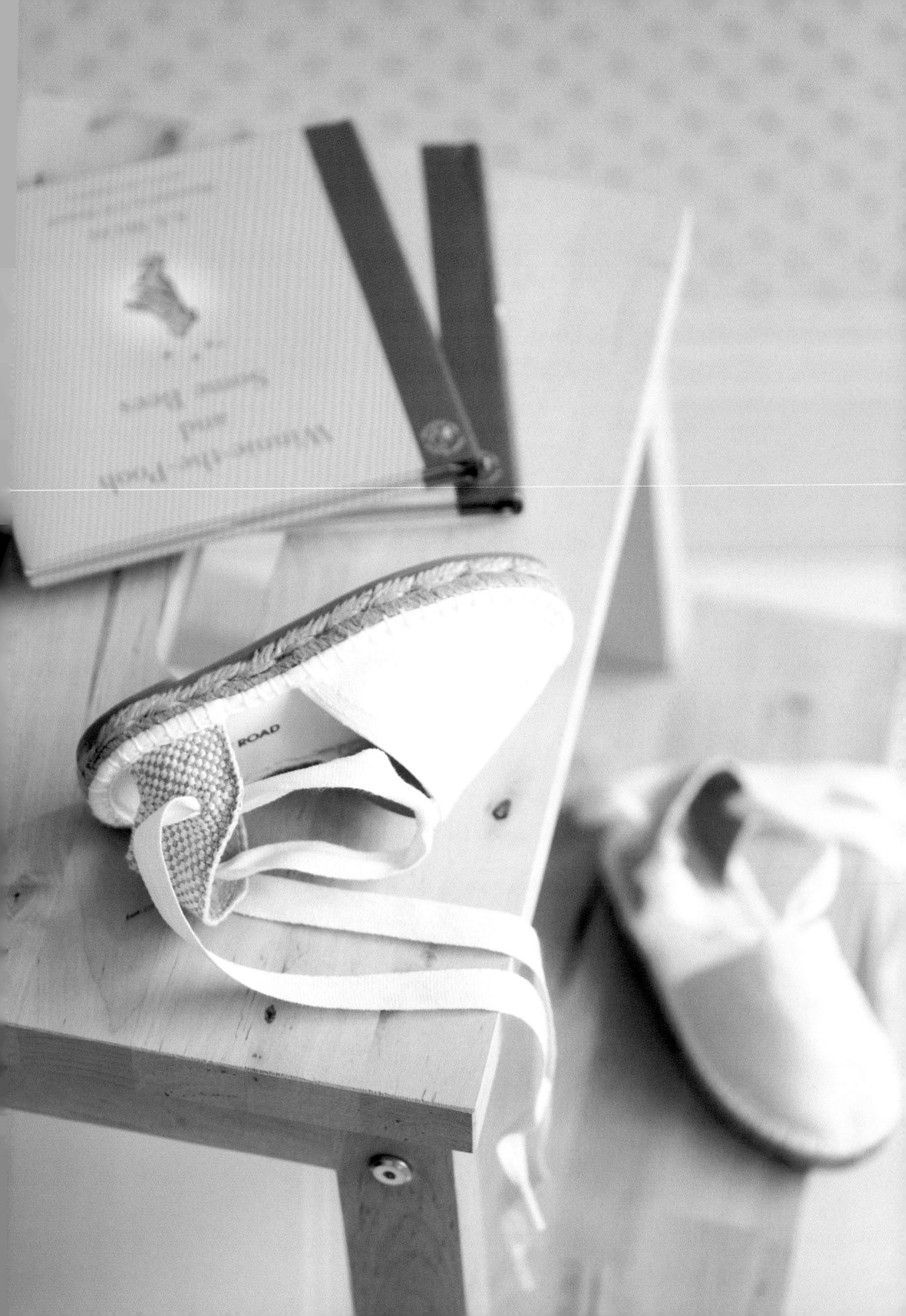

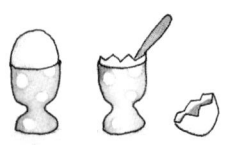

peach and **mango** smoothies

PREPARATION TIME 5 MINUTES MAKES 2 CUPS

1 small frozen mango (300g),
  chopped coarsely

⅓ cup (80ml) peach nectar

1 cup (250ml) milk

1 Blend or process
ingredients until smooth.

TIP You can use apricot nectar
instead of the peach, if you prefer.

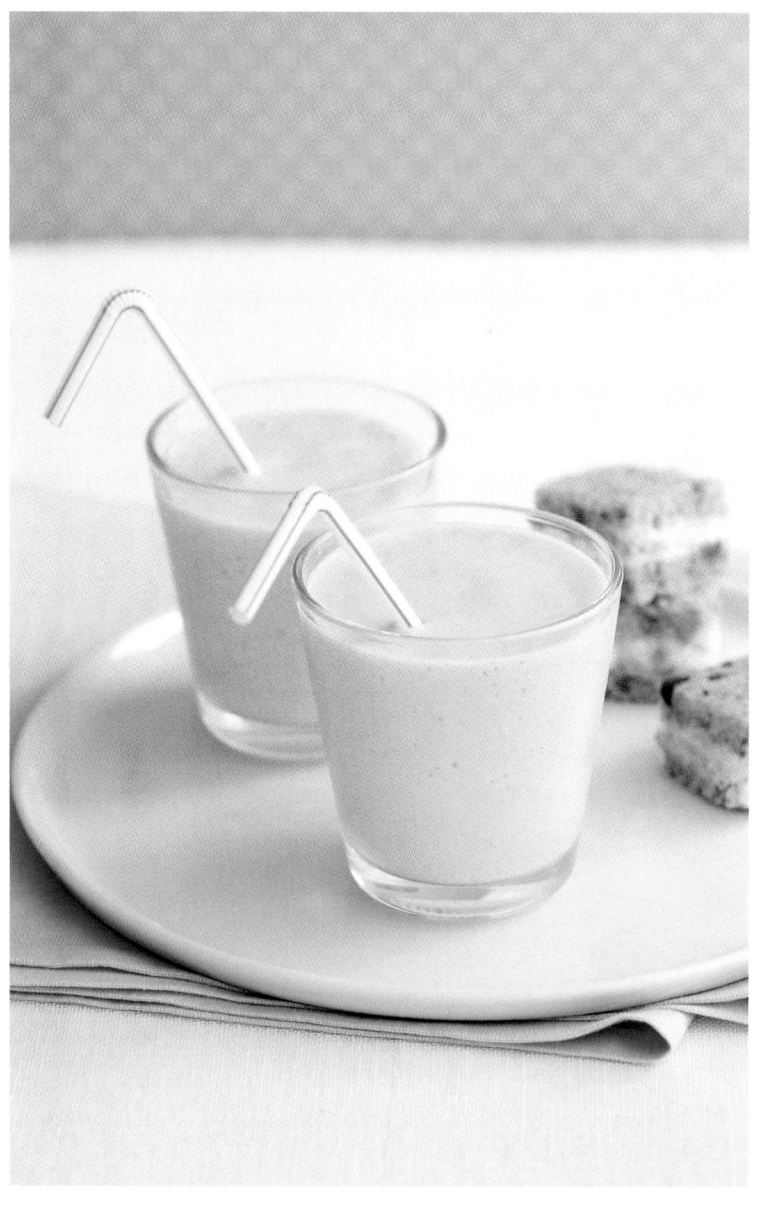

pancakes

PREPARATION TIME **5 MINUTES**
(PLUS STANDING TIME)
COOKING TIME **15 MINUTES** MAKES **10**

1 cup (150g) plain flour
1 egg
1¼ cups (310ml) milk

1 Sift flour into medium bowl; gradually whisk in combined egg and milk until smooth. Cover; stand 30 minutes. Transfer to medium jug.

2 Heat lightly oiled non-stick 14cm frying or pancake pan. Pour 2 tablespoons of the batter into pan; swirl to coat base of pan. Cook pancake, uncovered, until bubbles appear on surface. Turn pancake; cook, uncovered, until browned lightly. Repeat with remaining batter.

3 Serve pancakes plain or with a squeeze of lemon juice and a little sugar for the rest of the family.

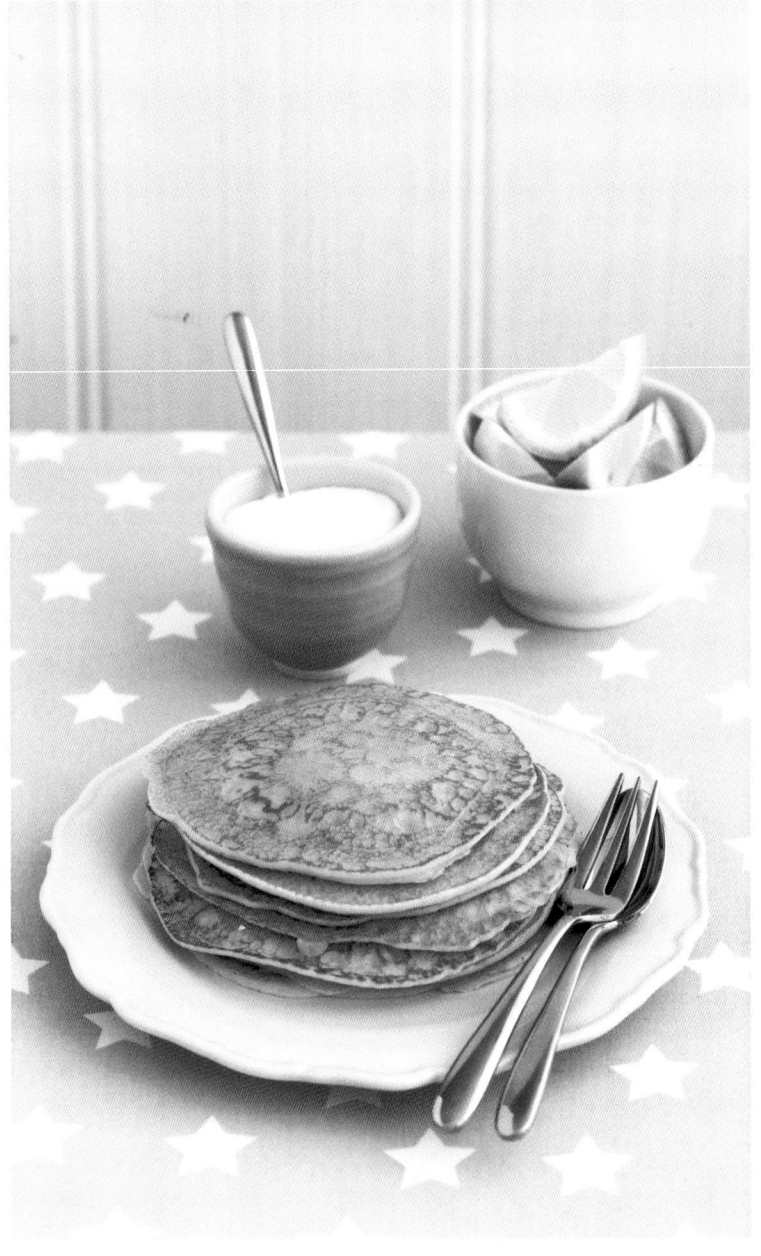

TIP Freeze any leftover pancakes, individually wrapped, for up to 1 month.

pasta **shells** with ricotta and tomato **sauce**

PREPARATION TIME **15 MINUTES**   COOKING TIME **25 MINUTES**   SERVES **4**

1 tablespoon olive oil

1 small brown onion (80g), chopped finely

1 medium carrot (120g), grated coarsely

1 clove garlic, crushed

1 tablespoon tomato paste

700g bottled tomato pasta sauce

1 cup (250ml) water

1 cup (120g) frozen peas

375g medium pasta shells

2 tablespoons finely chopped fresh flat-leaf parsley

200g ricotta cheese

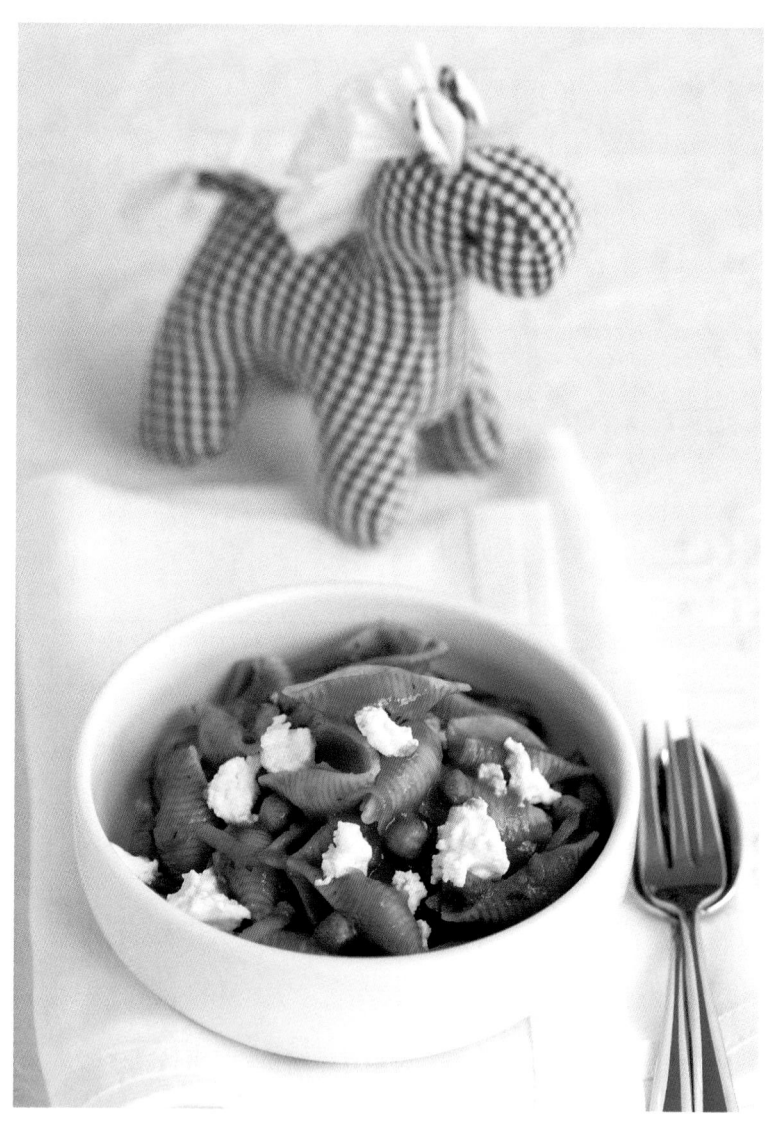

1 Heat oil in large frying pan; cook onion, carrot and garlic, stirring, until vegetables soften. Add paste; cook, stirring, 1 minute. Add sauce and the water; bring to a boil. Reduce heat; simmer, uncovered, 15 minutes. Add peas; simmer, uncovered, about 5 minutes or until sauce thickens slightly.

2 Meanwhile, cook pasta in large saucepan of boiling water, uncovered, until tender; drain.

3 Combine tomato sauce, pasta and parsley in large bowl. Divide among serving bowls; sprinkle with cheese.

TIP Leftover pasta can be frozen for up to 3 months.

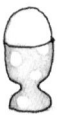

lentil patties

PREPARATION TIME 20 MINUTES

COOKING TIME 20 MINUTES MAKES 12

¼ cup (50g) red lentils

1 medium potato (200g),
   chopped coarsely

¼ cup (30g) frozen peas

½ small carrot (35g),
   grated coarsely

½ small brown onion (40g),
   grated finely

½ cup (50g) packaged
   breadcrumbs

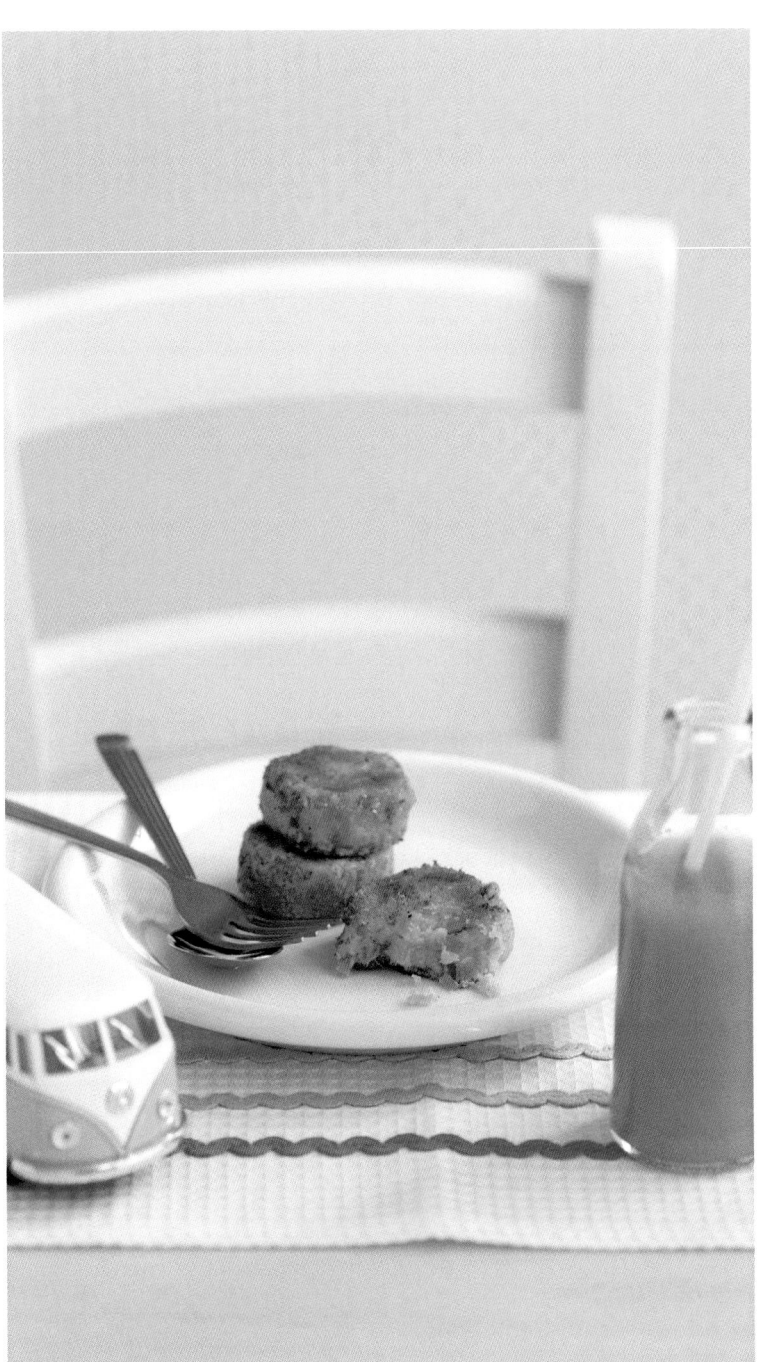

1 Cook lentils in small saucepan
   of boiling water, uncovered,
   about 10 minutes or until
   tender; drain.

2 Meanwhile, boil, steam or
   microwave potato and peas,
   separately, until tender; drain.
   Mash potato and peas in
   medium bowl.

3 Add lentils with carrot, onion
   and half of the breadcrumbs
   to potato mixture; using hand,
   mix to combine. Shape mixture
   into 12 patties.

4 Coat patties with remaining
   breadcrumbs; cook patties,
   uncovered, in large heated
   lightly oiled non-stick frying
   pan about 10 minutes or until
   patties are browned both sides
   and heated through.

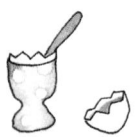

vegetable cakes

PREPARATION TIME 15 MINUTES

COOKING TIME 10 MINUTES MAKES 4

1 tablespoon olive oil

¼ cup (60g) coarsely grated potato

2 tablespoons finely chopped red capsicum

2 tablespoons finely chopped mushrooms

2 eggs, beaten lightly

1 tablespoon coarsely grated swiss cheese

1 Heat oil in medium frying pan; cook potato, stirring, until tender. Add capsicum and mushrooms; cook, stirring, until capsicum softens. Cool 10 minutes.

2 Combine potato mixture in small bowl with egg and cheese.

3 Place four oiled egg rings in medium heated lightly oiled non-stick frying pan; divide potato mixture among rings. Cook, uncovered, over low heat 5 minutes. Using egg slide, turn rings; cook, uncovered, until cakes set.

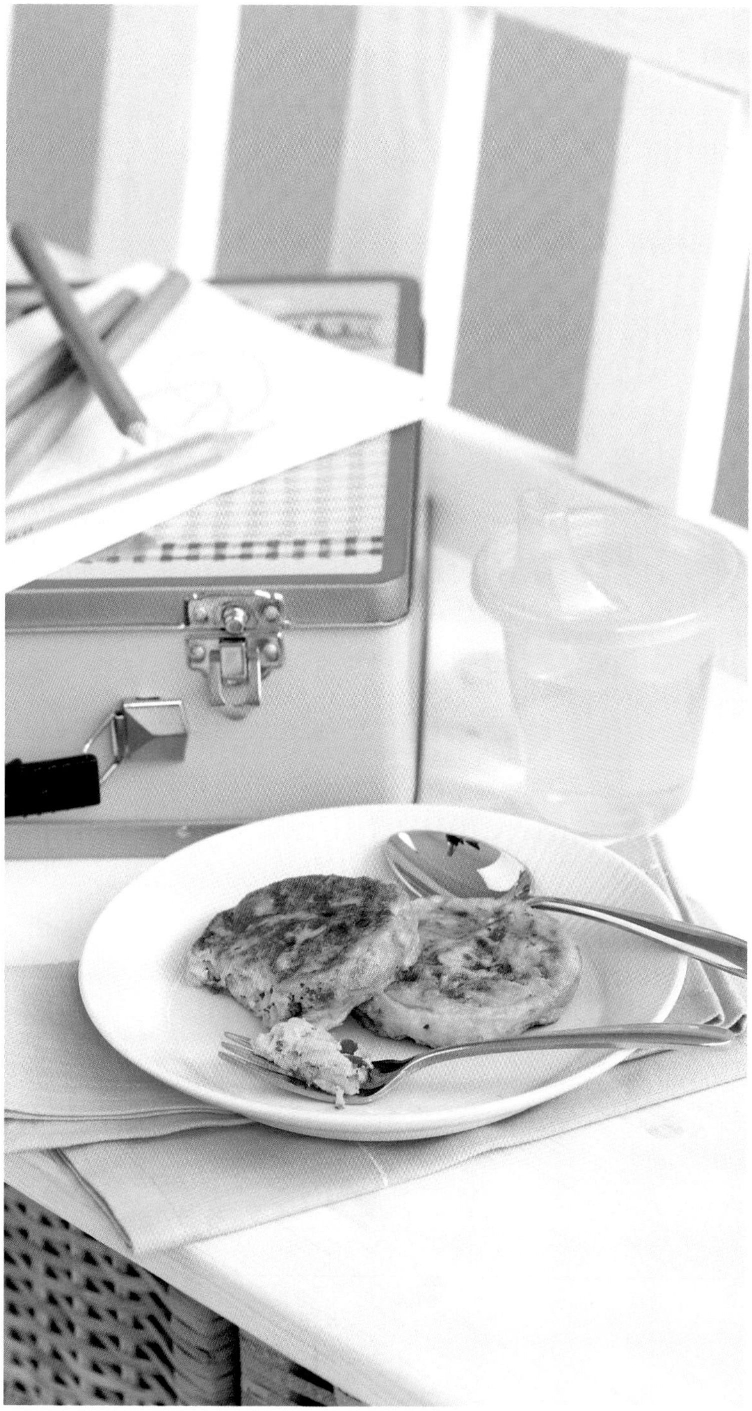

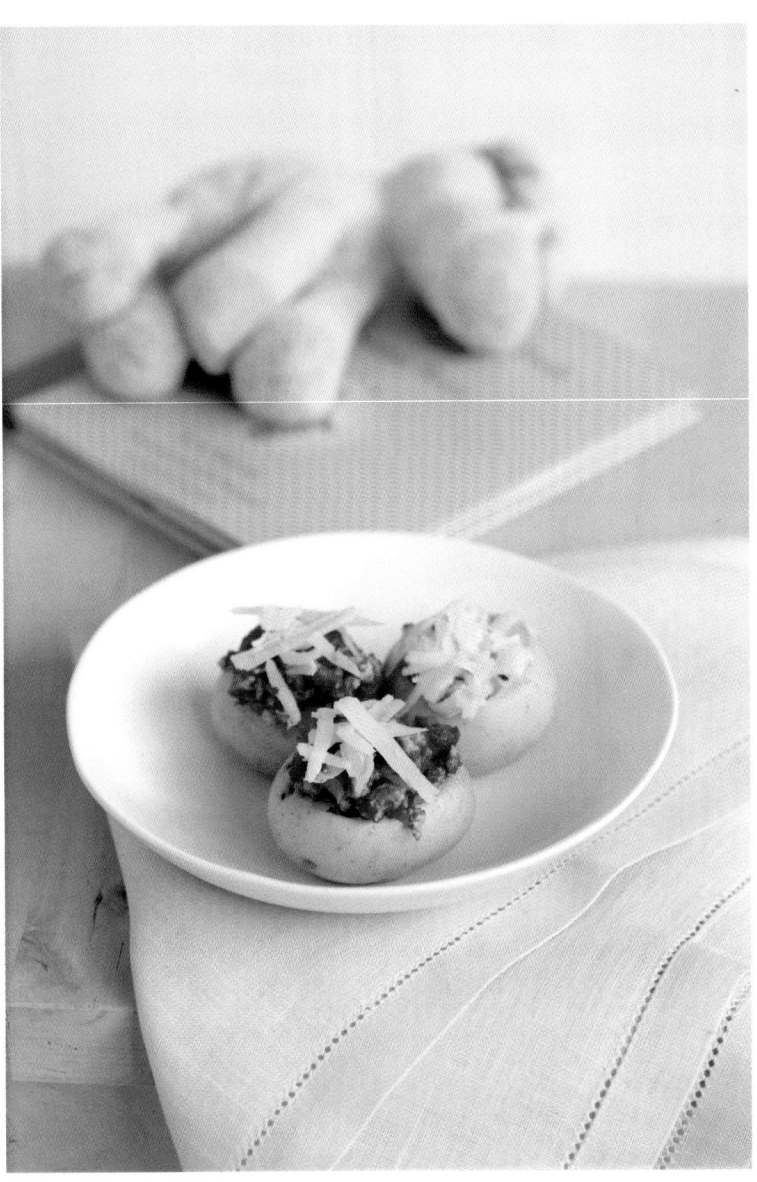

stuffed potatoes

PREPARATION TIME **15 MINUTES**
COOKING TIME **20 MINUTES** MAKES **12**

12 baby potatoes (480g)

1 teaspoon olive oil

½ small brown onion (40g), chopped finely

½ small carrot (35g), grated coarsely

100g chicken mince

½ cup (125ml) tomato purée

1 tablespoon coarsely grated parmesan

1 Boil, steam or microwave potatoes until tender; drain.

2 Meanwhile, heat oil in small frying pan; cook onion, stirring, until soft. Add carrot and mince; cook, stirring, about 5 minutes or until mince is browned and cooked through.

3 Add tomato purée; bring to a boil. Reduce heat; simmer, uncovered, about 5 minutes or until liquid evaporates.

4 Cut shallow slice from top of each potato; using teaspoon, carefully scoop out about two-thirds of the flesh. Spoon filling into potatoes; sprinkle with cheese.

TIP Make a little mashed potato out of scooped-out potato flesh.

vegetarian stuffing

Heat 1 teaspoon olive oil in small frying pan; cook 1 coarsely grated small zucchini (90g) and 3 coarsely grated yellow patty-pan squash (90g), stirring, until softened. Add ⅓ cup (80ml) milk; bring to a boil. Reduce heat; simmer, uncovered, about 5 minutes or until liquid evaporates. Stir in 2 tablespoons coarsely grated cheddar.

rissoles

PREPARATION TIME 15 MINUTES

COOKING TIME 30 MINUTES MAKES 30

500g beef mince

1 small carrot (70g), grated coarsely

1 small zucchini (90g),
    grated coarsely

½ small brown onion (40g),
    grated coarsely

½ cup (35g) stale breadcrumbs

1 tablespoon tomato sauce

2 teaspoons soy sauce

1 tablespoon olive oil

TANGY SAUCE

2 tablespoons tomato sauce

2 tablespoons barbecue sauce

2 teaspoons soy sauce

2 teaspoons worcestershire sauce

1 clove garlic, crushed

¼ cup (60ml) water

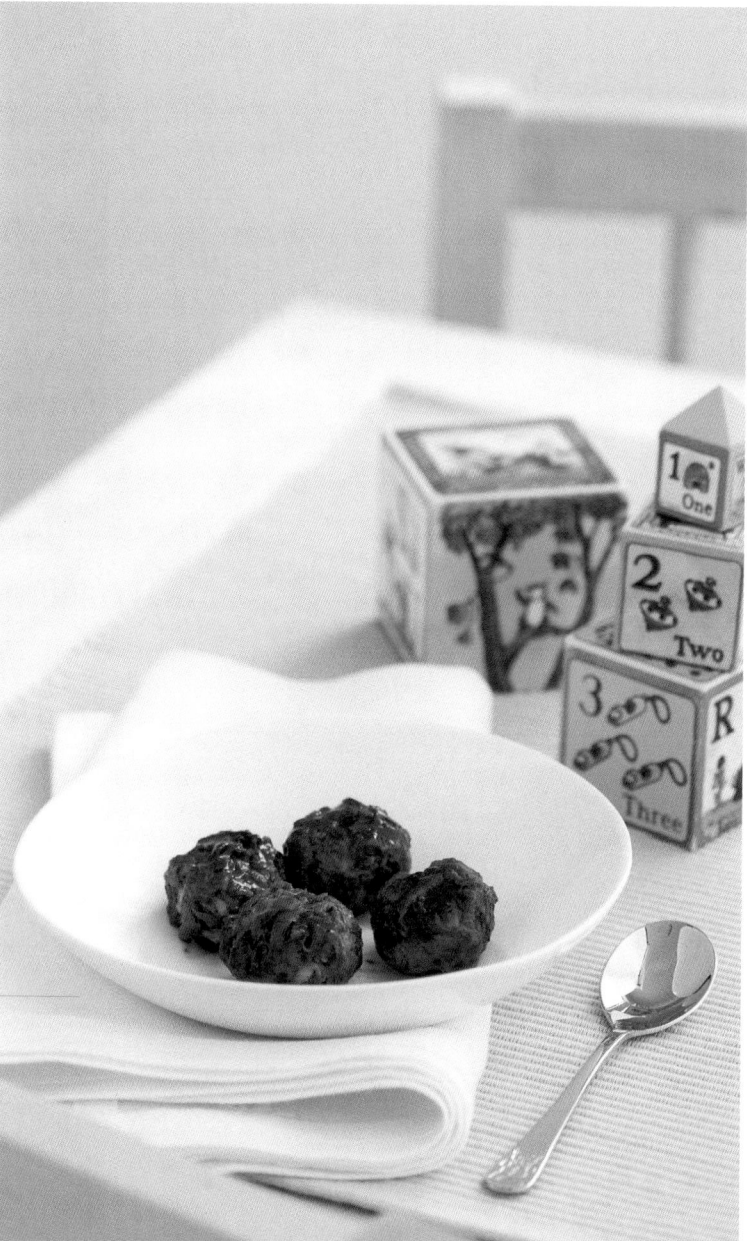

1 Preheat oven to moderate.
2 Using hand, combine mince, carrot, zucchini, onion, breadcrumbs and sauces in large bowl. Roll level tablespoons of the mixture into balls.
3 Combine ingredients for tangy sauce in small bowl.
4 Heat oil in large non-stick frying pan; cook rissoles, in batches, until browned all over. Transfer to medium shallow baking dish; cover with tangy sauce. Cook, uncovered, in moderate oven about 20 minutes or until rissoles are cooked through.

TIPS To make gluten free, replace breadcrumbs with half a cup of cooked rice.

Uncooked rissoles can be frozen for up to 2 months.

Chicken, pork or lamb mince can be used instead of beef.

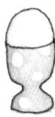

easy lamb and bean casserole

PREPARATION TIME 15 MINUTES COOKING TIME 2 HOURS MAKES 3 CUPS

2 teaspoons olive oil

1 clove garlic, crushed

1 small brown onion (80g),
    chopped coarsely

1 small carrot (70g), chopped finely

1 trimmed celery stick (100g),
    chopped finely

250g diced lamb shoulder

2 cups (500ml) chicken stock

425g can diced tomatoes

300g can mixed beans, drained

¼ cup finely chopped fresh
    flat leaf parsley

1 Heat oil in medium
   saucepan; cook garlic, onion,
   carrot and celery, stirring,
   until onion softens.

2 Add lamb, stock and
   undrained tomatoes; bring
   to a boil. Reduce heat;
   simmer, covered, 1 hour.
   Add beans; simmer,
   uncovered, about 1 hour
   or until lamb is tender.
   Stir in parsley.

TIP Freeze any remaining
casserole, covered, for up
to 3 months.

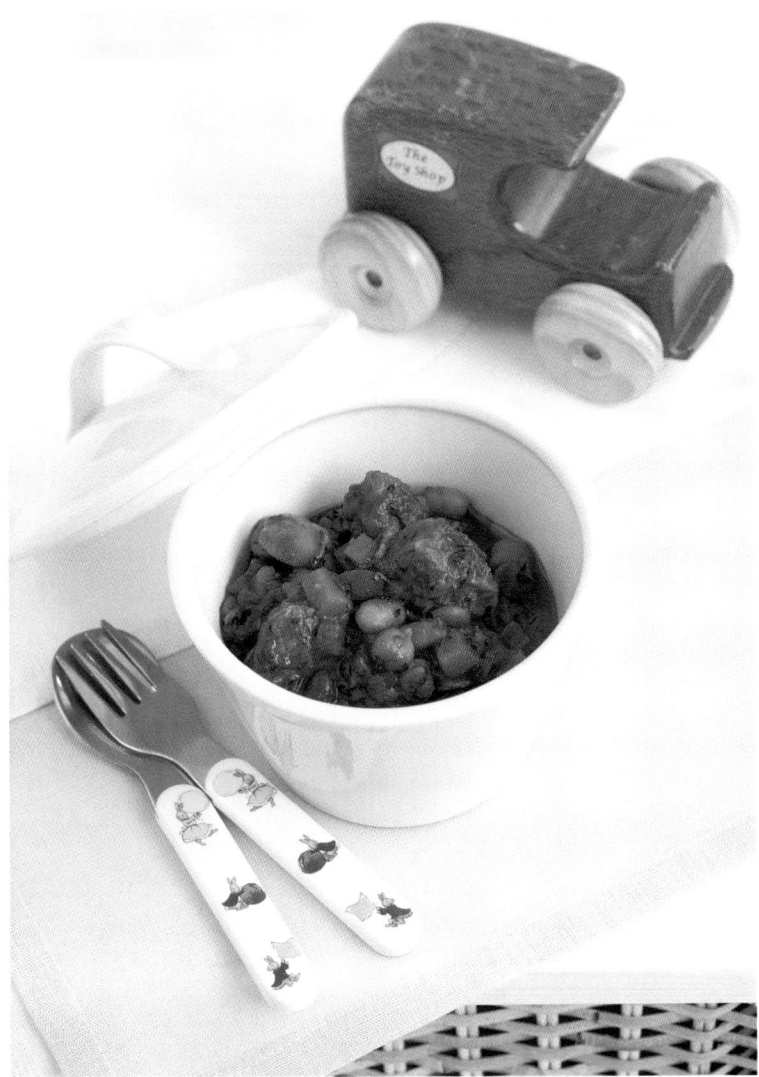

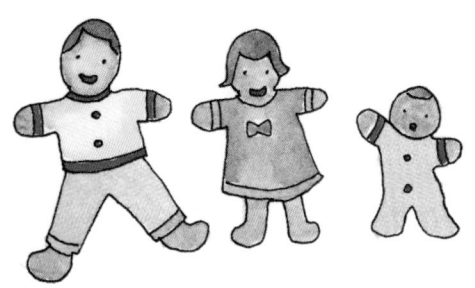

FAMILY MEALS

Recipes that appeal to adults *and* toddlers are a boon for the cook of the family. Accordingly, the flavours, spice levels and foods used in this chapter are for meals suitable for all. Look out for the "toddler tip" following some recipes for suggestions on how the dish can be slightly amended for kids.

asian grilled chicken with green beans

PREPARATION TIME **15 MINUTES (PLUS REFRIGERATION TIME)** COOKING TIME **20 MINUTES** SERVES **4**

2 tablespoons hoisin sauce

2 tablespoons lime juice

1 tablespoon soy sauce

2cm piece fresh ginger (10g), grated

1 clove garlic, crushed

6 chicken thigh fillets (660g), halved

400g green beans, trimmed

2 teaspoons peanut oil

2 green onions, sliced thinly

2 tablespoons oyster sauce

1 Combine hoisin, juice, soy, ginger and garlic in medium bowl, add chicken; turn chicken to coat in marinade. Cover; refrigerate 1 hour.

2 Cook drained chicken on heated oiled grill plate (or grill or barbecue) until cooked through.

3 Meanwhile, boil, steam or microwave beans until just tender; drain. Heat oil in medium frying pan; cook beans, onion and oyster sauce, stirring, until heated through.

4 Serve chicken and beans with steamed jasmine rice, if desired.

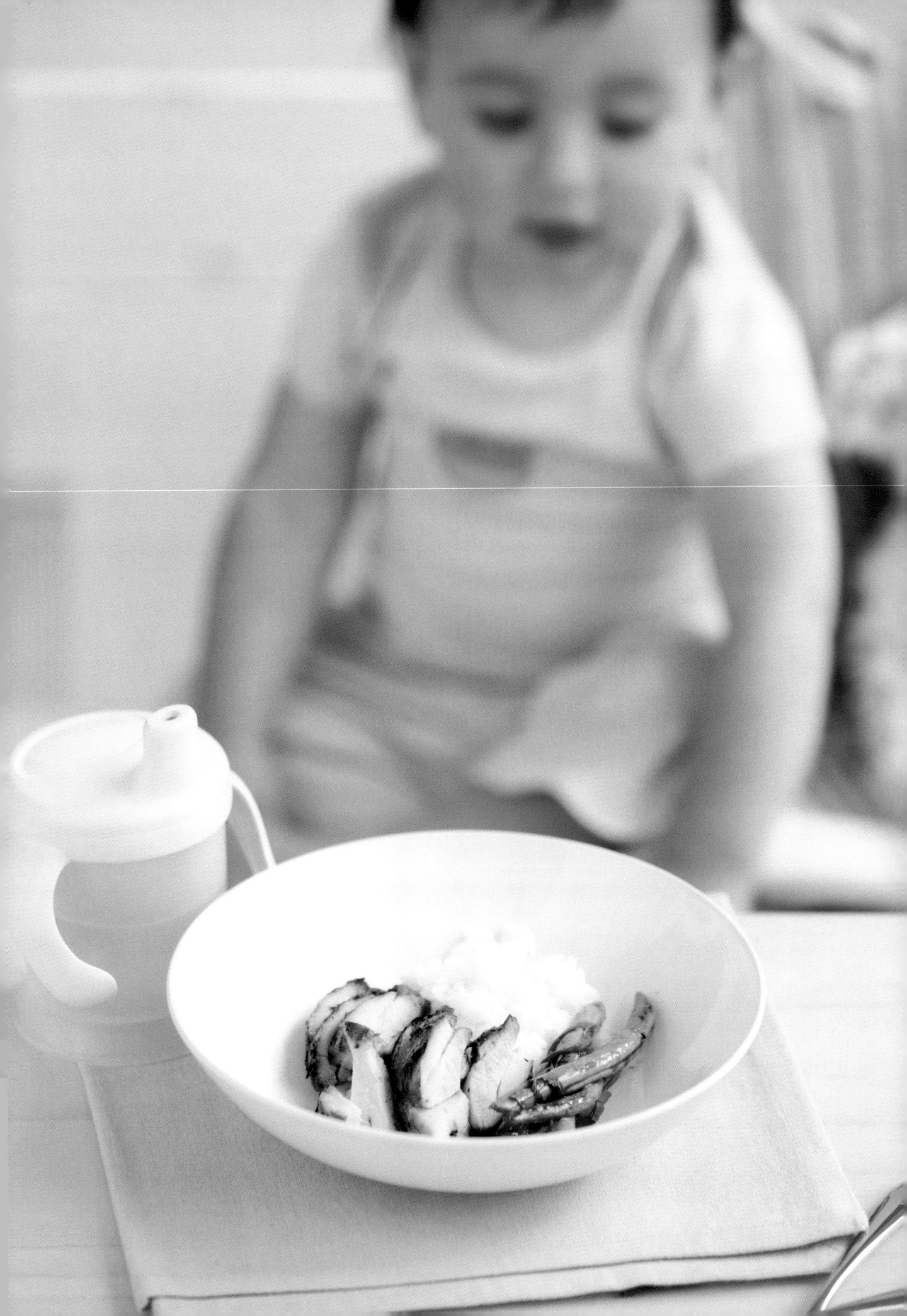

broccoli and cheese frittata with tomato salad

PREPARATION TIME 15 MINUTES   COOKING TIME 30 MINUTES   SERVES 4

400g broccoli

1 cup (120g) coarsely
  grated cheddar

½ cup (40g) coarsely
  grated parmesan

7 eggs

⅓ cup (80ml) cream

TOMATO SALAD

500g cherry tomatoes, halved

200g yellow teardrop
  tomatoes, halved

½ cup loosely packed baby
  basil leaves

2 tablespoons balsamic vinegar

1 tablespoon olive oil

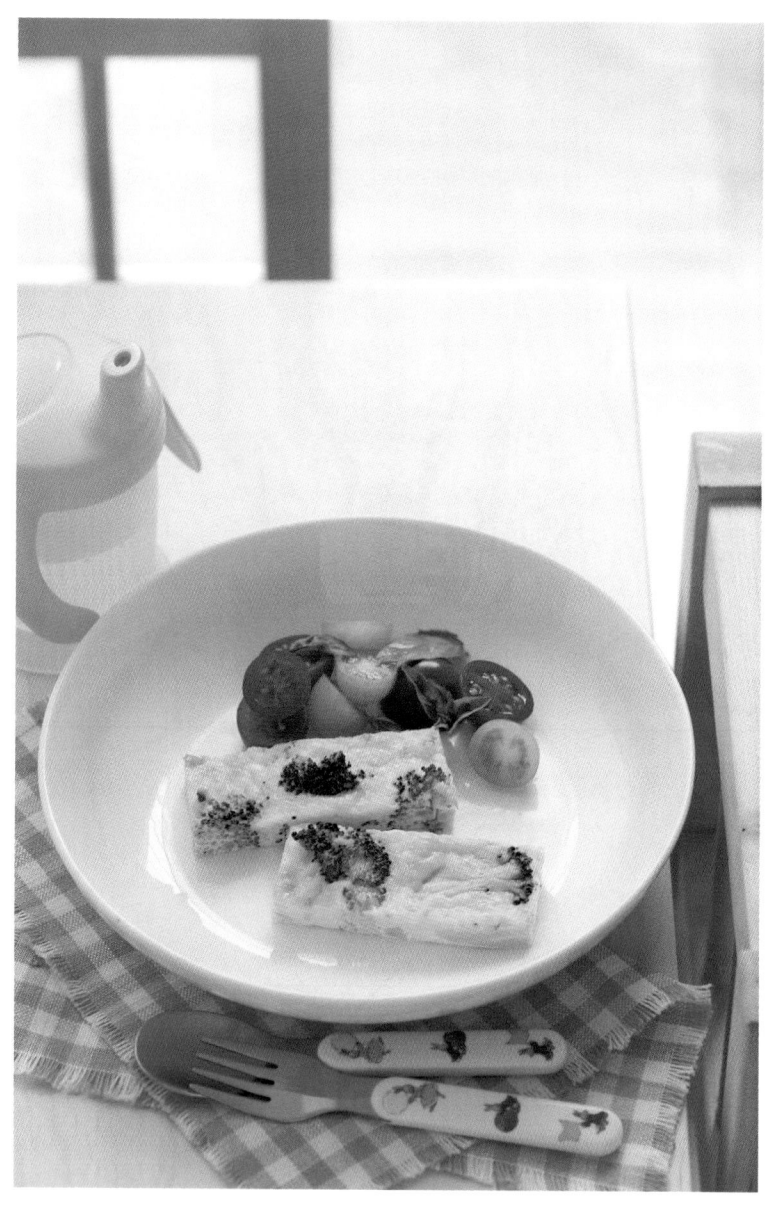

1 Preheat oven to moderate.
   Grease 20cm x 30cm
   lamington pan. Line base
   and sides with baking paper.
2 Discard broccoli stalks; thinly
   slice florets vertically. Place
   broccoli in large saucepan of
   boiling water; return to a boil,
   drain. Rinse under cold
   water; drain. Pat dry with
   absorbent paper.
3 Layer broccoli and combined
   cheeses in prepared pan
   then pour over combined
   eggs and cream. Cook,
   uncovered, in moderate oven
   about 25 minutes or until
   frittata sets. Cool 5 minutes.
4 Meanwhile, combine
   ingredients for tomato
   salad in medium bowl.
5 Serve frittata with salad.

TODDLER TIP Don't dress
toddler's salad portion.

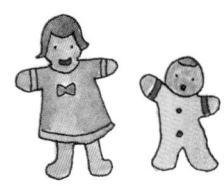

roast butterflied chicken with mash and fresh corn

PREPARATION TIME **20 MINUTES** COOKING TIME **45 MINUTES** SERVES **4**

1.6kg chicken

30g butter, softened

1 teaspoon finely chopped
fresh thyme

2 teaspoons finely grated
lemon rind

3 trimmed corn cobs
(750g), quartered

CREAMY MASH

800g potatoes, chopped coarsely

⅔ cup (160ml) warm milk

20g butter

1 Preheat oven to hot.

2 Using kitchen scissors, cut
along both sides of backbone
of chicken; discard backbone.
Place chicken, skin-side up,
on board; using heel of hand,
press down on breastbone
to flatten chicken.

3 Combine butter, thyme and
rind in small bowl. Loosen
skin of chicken by sliding
fingers between skin and
meat at the neck joint. Push
butter mixture under skin.

4 Place chicken on lightly
oiled wire rack in large
shallow baking dish; roast,
uncovered, in hot oven
about 45 minutes or until
chicken is cooked through.

5 Meanwhile, make creamy
mash. Boil, steam, or
microwave corn until
tender; drain.

6 Serve chicken with corn
and creamy mash.

creamy mash Boil, steam or
microwave potato until tender;
drain. Mash potato in large
bowl with milk and butter.

TODDLER TIP Remove kernels
from one corn cob quarter and
chop them with a small piece of
chicken meat. Serve with a few
tablespoons of creamy mash.

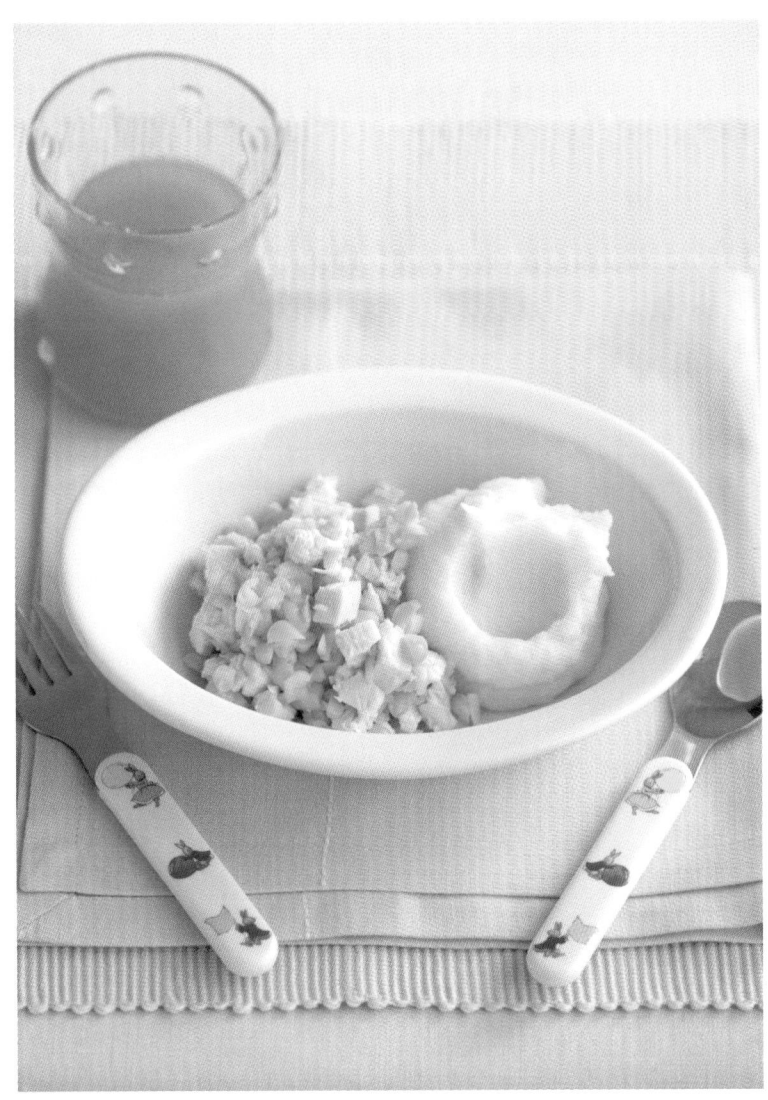

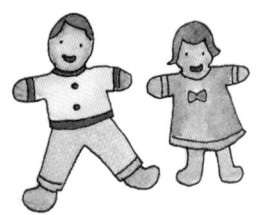

macaroni cheese with spinach and bacon

PREPARATION TIME **20 MINUTES** COOKING TIME **50 MINUTES** SERVES **6**

375g elbow macaroni

300g spinach, trimmed

1 medium brown onion (150g),
chopped finely

4 bacon rashers (280g), rind
removed, chopped finely

50g butter

⅓ cup (50g) plain flour

1 litre (4 cups) hot milk

1½ cups (180g) coarsely
grated cheddar

½ cup (35g) stale breadcrumbs

1 Preheat oven to
moderately hot.

2 Cook pasta in large saucepan
of boiling water, uncovered,
until just tender; drain.

3 Meanwhile, steam or
microwave spinach until
wilted; drain. Rinse under
cold water; drain. Squeeze
as much liquid as possible
from spinach; chop coarsely.

4 Cook onion and bacon,
stirring, in medium saucepan
until onion softens. Transfer
to large bowl.

5 Melt butter in same pan,
add flour; cook, stirring,
until mixture thickens and
bubbles. Gradually add milk;
stir until mixture boils and
thickens. Remove from heat;
stir in cheese.

6 Combine pasta, spinach
and cheese sauce in bowl
with onion mixture. Pour into
greased shallow 2.5-litre
(10 cup) flameproof casserole
dish; top with breadcrumbs.

7 Cook, uncovered, in
moderately hot oven about
30 minutes. Place dish
under preheated grill to
brown lightly.

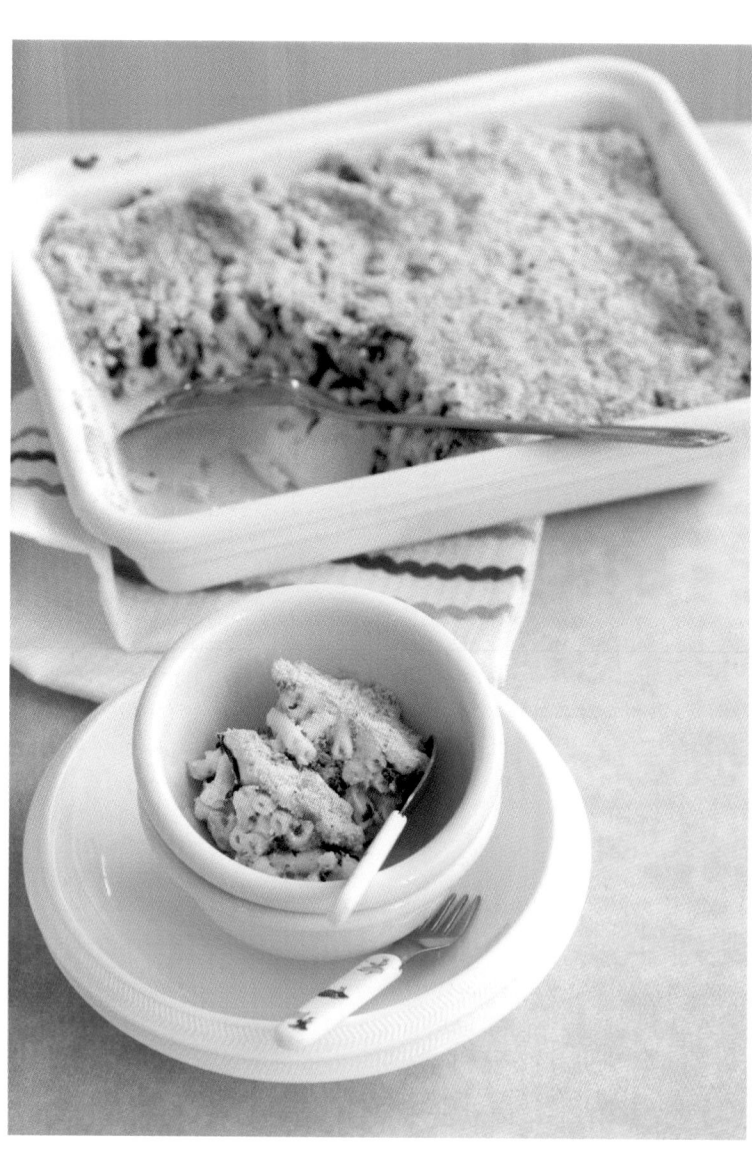

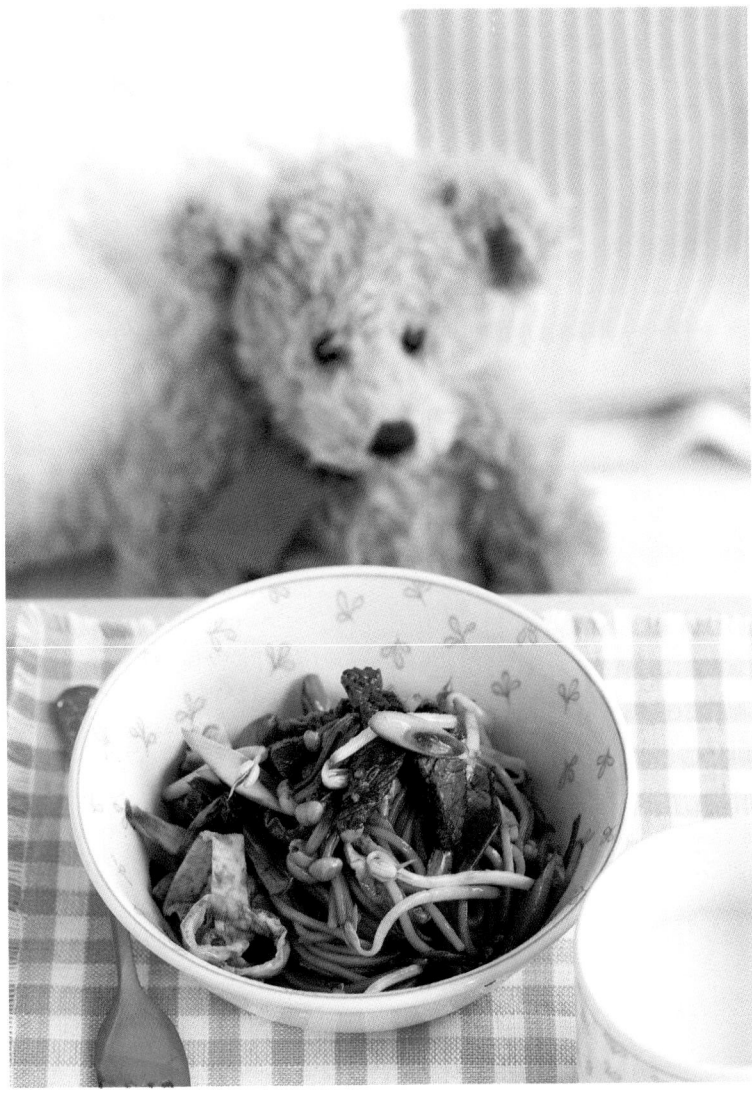

stir-fried beef with hokkien noodles

PREPARATION TIME 15 MINUTES   COOKING TIME 15 MINUTES   SERVES 4

2 tablespoons peanut oil

2 eggs, beaten lightly

400g thin hokkien noodles

2 cloves garlic, crushed

600g beef rump steak,
  sliced thinly

¼ cup (60ml) kecap manis

1 tablespoon fish sauce

1 tablespoon oyster sauce

1½ cups (120g) bean sprouts

100g enoki mushrooms, trimmed

150g oyster mushrooms,
  chopped coarsely

4 green onions, sliced thickly

1 Heat half of the oil in wok; cook egg over medium heat, swirling wok to make a thin omelette. Transfer to board; when cool, roll into cigar shape, slice thinly.

2 Place noodles in medium heatproof bowl; cover with boiling water, separate with fork, drain.

3 Heat remaining oil in same wok; stir-fry garlic and beef, in batches, until beef is browned. Return beef mixture to wok with noodles, sauces, sprouts, mushrooms and onion; stir-fry until heated through. Remove from heat; add sliced omelette, toss gently to combine.

TODDLER TIP Omit the green onions, if desired. Cut toddler portion of beef into small pieces to serve.

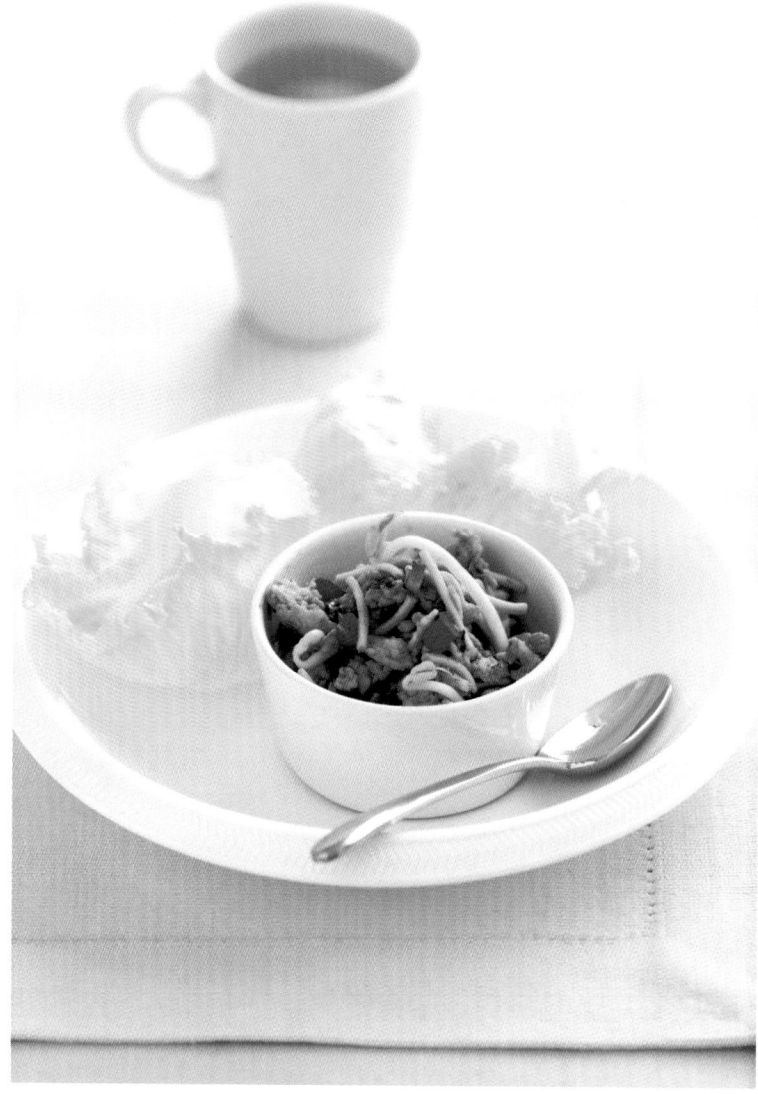

chicken sang choy bow

PREPARATION TIME 15 MINUTES

COOKING TIME 15 MINUTES SERVES 4

1 tablespoon peanut oil

700g chicken mince

1 small red capsicum (150g), chopped finely

150g mushrooms, chopped finely

1 clove garlic, crushed

3 green onions, chopped finely

2 tablespoons oyster sauce

2 tablespoons soy sauce

2 tablespoons hoisin sauce

1 teaspoon sesame oil

2 cups (160g) bean sprouts

100g packet fried crunchy noodles

8 large iceberg lettuce leaves

2 green onions, sliced thinly, extra

1 Heat peanut oil in wok; stir-fry chicken until changed in colour.

2 Add capsicum, mushrooms and garlic; stir-fry until vegetables are just tender.

3 Add chopped onion, sauces and sesame oil; stir-fry until chicken is cooked through. Remove from heat; stir in sprouts and noodles.

4 Divide lettuce leaves among serving plates. Spoon chicken mixture into leaves; sprinkle each with sliced onion.

TODDLER TIP Choose a small lettuce leaf; spoon chicken mixture into leaf without adding green onion then roll into small, tight cigar shape to be eaten by hand.

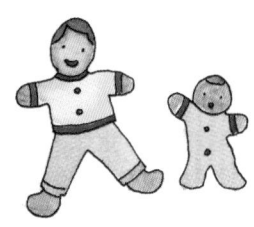

minestrone with meatballs

PREPARATION TIME **40 MINUTES** COOKING TIME **35 MINUTES** SERVES **4**

400g pork mince

1 teaspoon sweet paprika

1 egg, beaten lightly

1 medium brown onion (150g),
  chopped finely

¼ cup (70g) tomato paste

2 tablespoons olive oil

2 cloves garlic, crushed

2 medium carrots (240g), diced
  into 1cm pieces

1 trimmed celery stick (100g),
  diced into 1cm pieces

2 x 425g cans diced tomatoes

2 cups (500ml) chicken stock

2 cups (500ml) water

2 large zucchini (300g), diced
  into 1cm pieces

400g can borlotti beans,
  rinsed, drained

½ cup (110g) risoni

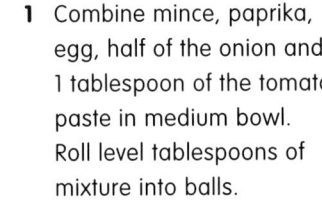

1 Combine mince, paprika, egg, half of the onion and 1 tablespoon of the tomato paste in medium bowl. Roll level tablespoons of mixture into balls.

2 Heat oil in large saucepan; cook meatballs, in batches, until browned. Cook garlic and remaining onion in same pan, stirring, until onion softens. Add carrot and celery; cook, stirring, until vegetables are just tender.

3 Add remaining paste to pan; cook, stirring, 1 minute. Add undrained tomatoes, stock and the water; bring to a boil.

4 Add zucchini, beans, risoni and meatballs; return to a boil. Reduce heat; simmer, covered, about 15 minutes or until meatballs are cooked through.

TODDLER TIP Purée a meatball and a toddler-size portion of the soup together.

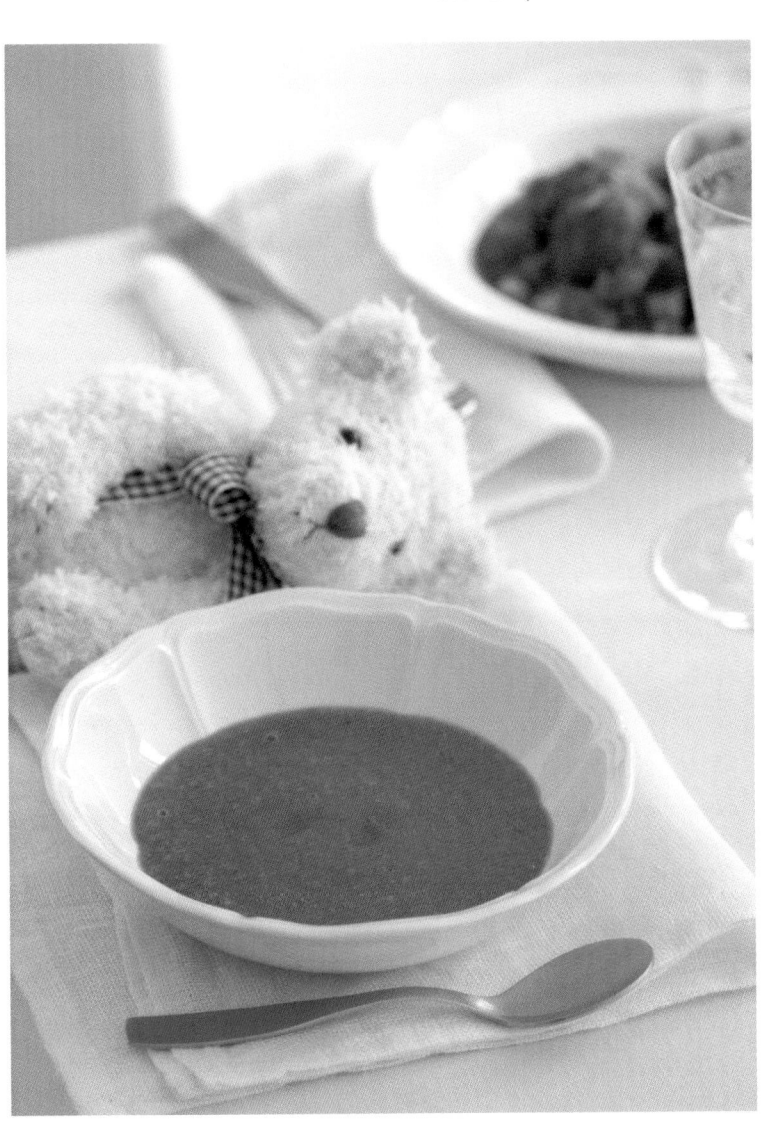

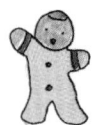

sausage pasta bake

PREPARATION TIME **15 MINUTES** COOKING TIME **45 MINUTES** SERVES **6**

6 thick beef sausages (480g)

375g penne

1 tablespoon olive oil

1 medium brown onion (150g),
chopped coarsely

1 small red capsicum (150g),
chopped coarsely

1 small yellow capsicum (150g),
chopped coarsely

1 large zucchini (150g), sliced thinly

200g mushrooms, quartered

¼ cup coarsely chopped
fresh basil

700g bottled tomato pasta sauce

¼ cup (60ml) water

1 cup (100g) coarsely
grated mozzarella

½ cup (40g) coarsely
grated parmesan

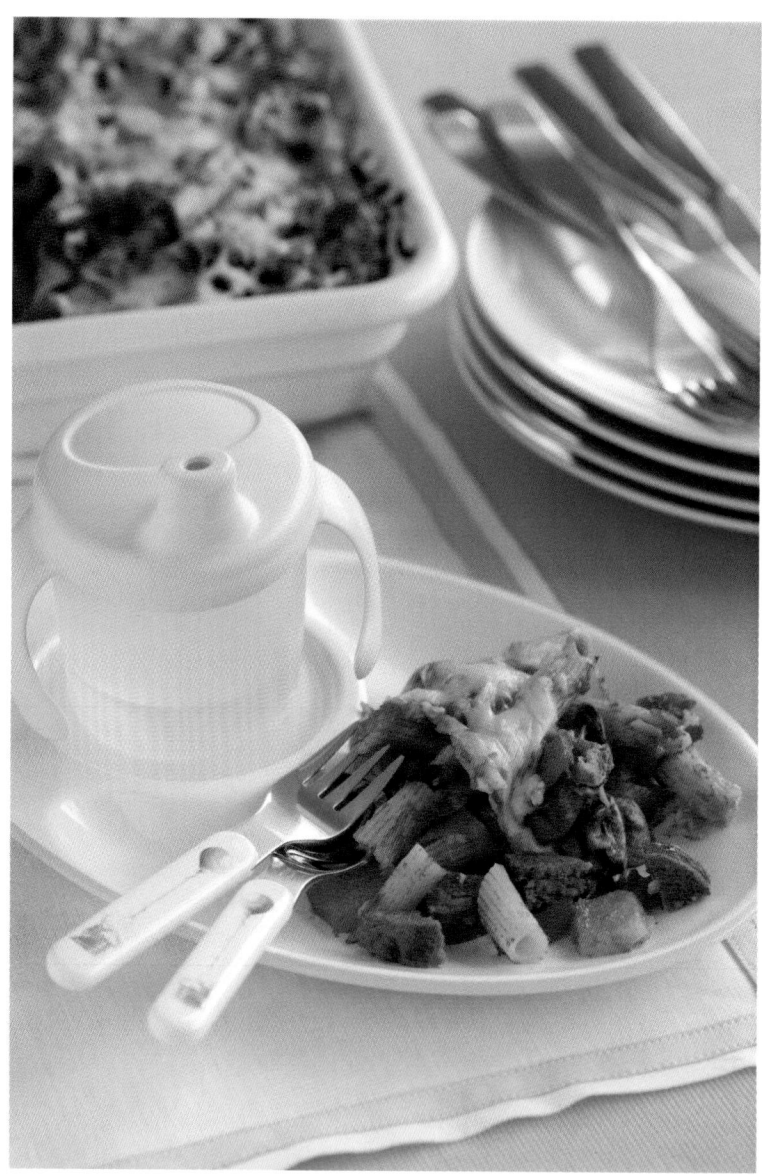

1 Preheat oven to
moderately hot.

2 Cook sausages in large
heated frying pan until
cooked through; cut into
1cm slices.

3 Meanwhile, cook pasta in
large saucepan of boiling
water, uncovered, until just
tender; drain.

4 Heat oil in same cleaned
frying pan; cook onion,
capsicums and zucchini,
stirring, until vegetables
are tender. Add mushrooms,
basil and pasta sauce;
bring to a boil. Reduce
heat; simmer, uncovered,
5 minutes.

5 Combine pasta in large
bowl with sliced sausage,
vegetable mixture and half
of the mozzarella.

6 Place in 2.5-litre (10 cup)
shallow baking dish; sprinkle
with combined remaining
cheeses. Bake, uncovered,
in moderately hot oven
about 25 minutes or until
browned lightly.

TODDLER TIP Chop toddler
portion of the bake into
bite-size pieces.

chicken and vegetable soup

PREPARATION TIME **10 MINUTES** COOKING TIME **20 MINUTES** SERVES **4**

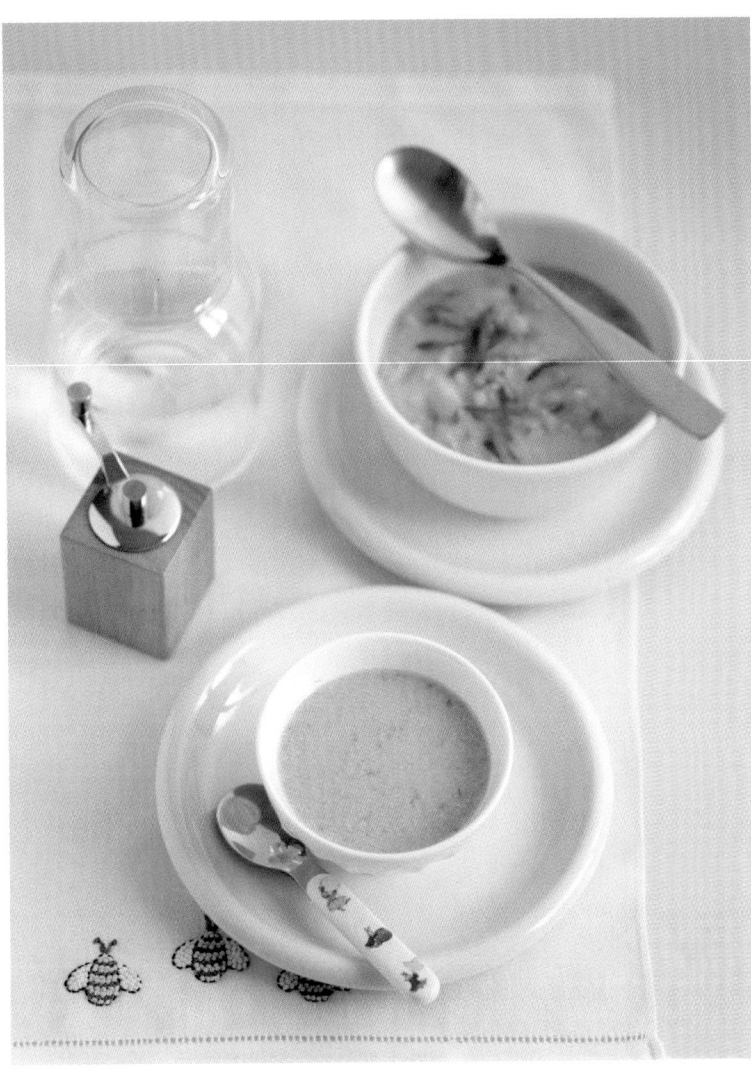

2 teaspoons vegetable oil

2 green onions, sliced thinly

1 clove garlic, crushed

2 cups (500ml) chicken stock

2 cups (500ml) water

350g chicken mince

1 tablespoon cornflour

¼ cup (60ml) water, extra

310g can creamed corn

1 cup (160g) fresh corn kernels

100g snow peas, trimmed, sliced thinly

1 egg, beaten lightly

1 Heat oil in large saucepan; cook onion and garlic, stirring, until onion softens. Add stock and the water; bring to a boil. Add chicken, reduce heat; simmer, stirring, about 5 minutes or until chicken is cooked through.

2 Blend cornflour and extra water in small jug; add to pan with creamed corn, corn kernels and snow peas. Cook, stirring, until mixture boils and thickens. Gradually add egg, in thin stream, to soup just before serving.

TODDLER TIP Purée toddler portion before adding egg.

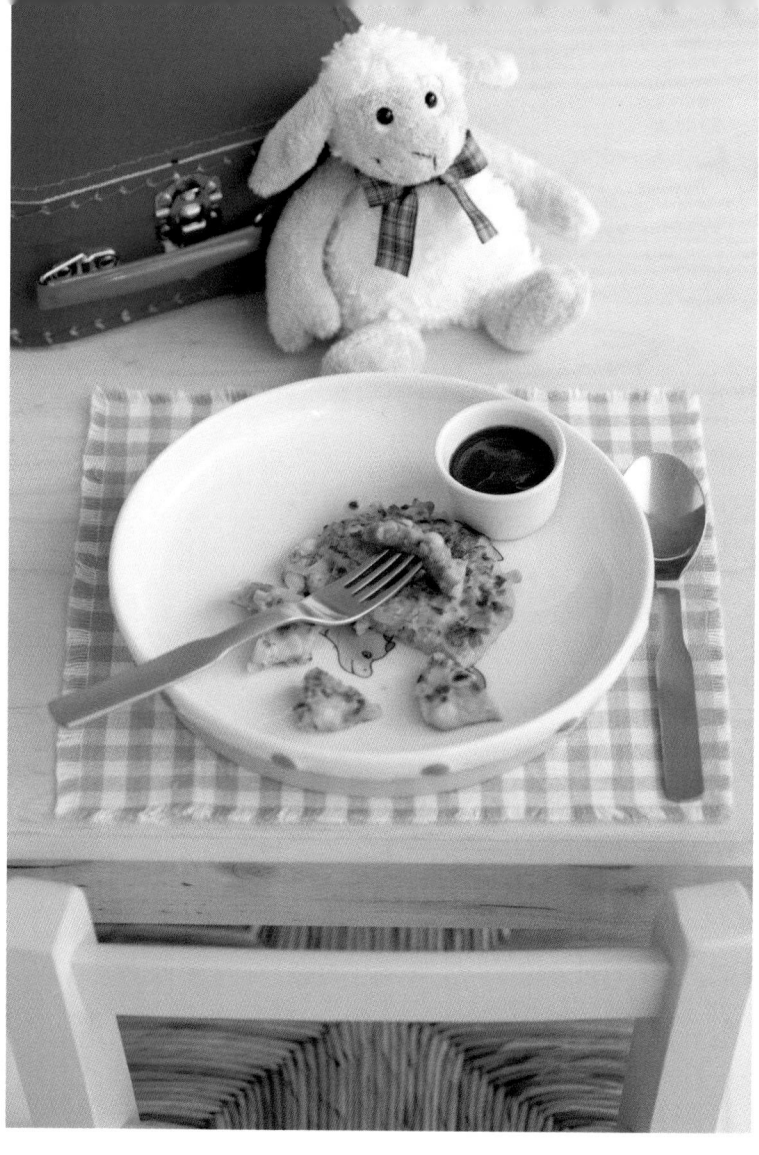

corn and bacon fritters

PREPARATION TIME 15 MINUTES COOKING TIME 20 MINUTES SERVES 4

You will need 2 fresh corn cobs for this recipe.

4 bacon rashers (280g), rind removed, chopped finely

2 cups (320g) fresh corn kernels

2 green onions, chopped finely

⅔ cup (100g) plain flour

½ teaspoon bicarbonate of soda

⅔ cup (160ml) buttermilk

2 eggs

125g can creamed corn

½ cup (125ml) sweet chilli sauce

1 Cook bacon in large non-stick frying pan until crisp. Add corn kernels and onion; cook, stirring, 2 minutes. Remove from heat.

2 Sift flour and soda into medium bowl. Make well in centre of flour mixture; gradually whisk in combined milk and eggs, whisking until batter is smooth. Stir in bacon mixture and creamed corn.

3 Pour ¼ cup batter into same heated oiled frying pan; using spatula, spread batter into round shape. Cook, two at a time, about 2 minutes each

side or until fritter is browned lightly and cooked through. Remove fritters from pan; cover to keep warm. Repeat process with remaining batter.

4 Divide fritters among serving plates; serve with sweet chilli sauce.

TODDLER TIP Serve toddler a small fritter with tomato sauce rather than sweet chilli sauce.

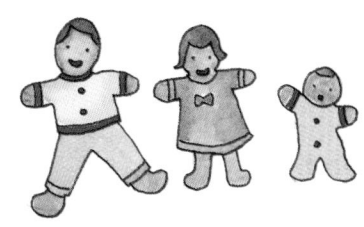

zucchini, pea and mint risotto

PREPARATION TIME **20 MINUTES**   COOKING TIME **45 MINUTES**   SERVES **4**

1 litre (4 cups) chicken stock

2 cups (500ml) water

40g butter

2 large zucchini (300g), halved, sliced thinly

1 clove garlic, crushed

1 small brown onion (80g), chopped finely

2 cups (400g) arborio rice

2 cups (240g) frozen peas, thawed

⅓ cup (25g) coarsely grated parmesan

1 tablespoon finely chopped fresh mint

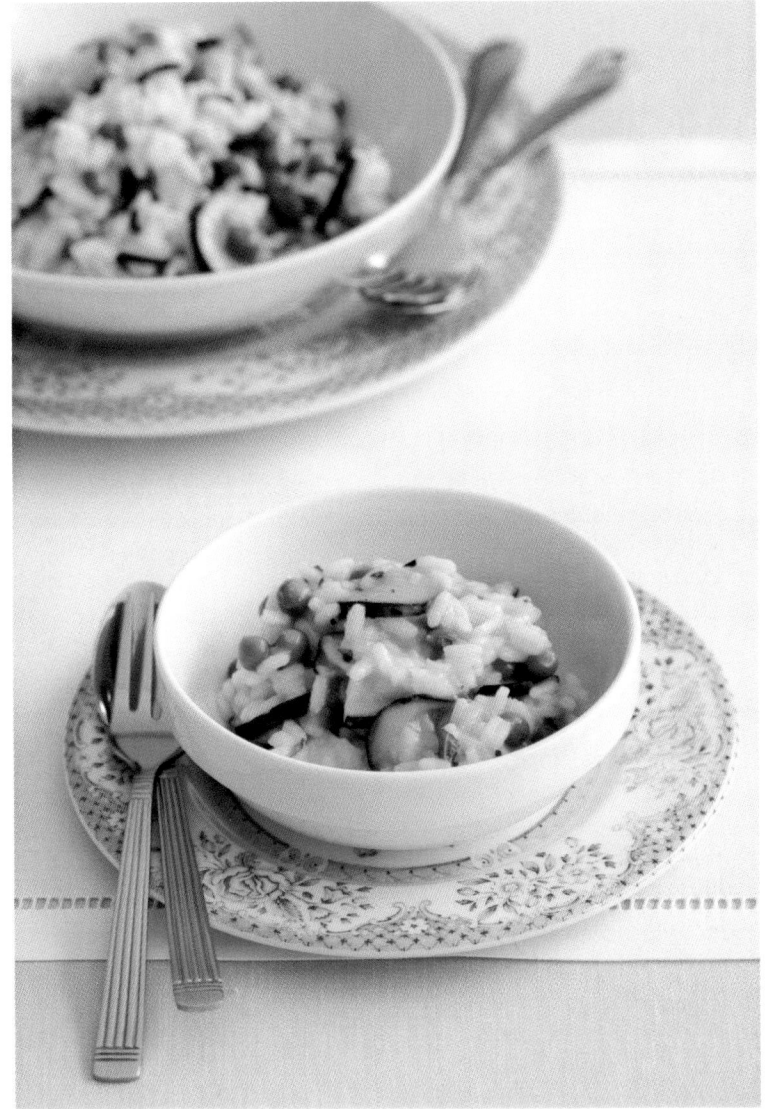

1 Combine stock and the water in medium saucepan; bring to a boil. Reduce heat; simmer, covered.

2 Meanwhile, melt butter in large saucepan; cook zucchini and garlic, stirring, until zucchini just softens. Remove from pan.

3 Cook onion in same pan, stirring, until softened. Add rice; stir to coat rice in onion mixture. Stir in 1 cup of the simmering stock mixture; cook, stirring, over low heat until liquid is absorbed. Continue adding stock mixture, in 1-cup batches, stirring, until liquid is absorbed after each addition. Total cooking time should be about 35 minutes or until rice is just tender.

4 Gently stir zucchini mixture and peas into risotto; cook, uncovered, until peas are tender. Remove from heat; stir in cheese and mint.

bolognese and spinach potato pie

PREPARATION TIME 25 MINUTES
COOKING TIME 1 HOUR 10 MINUTES
SERVES 6

This recipe is the perfect way to use any leftover bolognese sauce you may have from a previous meal (you'll need 3 cups).

1 tablespoon olive oil

1 small brown onion (80g), chopped finely

1 clove garlic, crushed

250g beef mince

1 small carrot (70g), grated coarsely

1 small red capsicum (150g), chopped finely

50g mushrooms, sliced thinly

2 tablespoons tomato paste

¼ cup (60ml) dry red wine

425g can crushed tomatoes

300g spinach, trimmed, chopped coarsely

5 medium potatoes (1.2kg)

40g unsalted butter

2 cloves garlic, crushed

2 eggs, beaten lightly

½ cup (50g) coarsely grated mozzarella

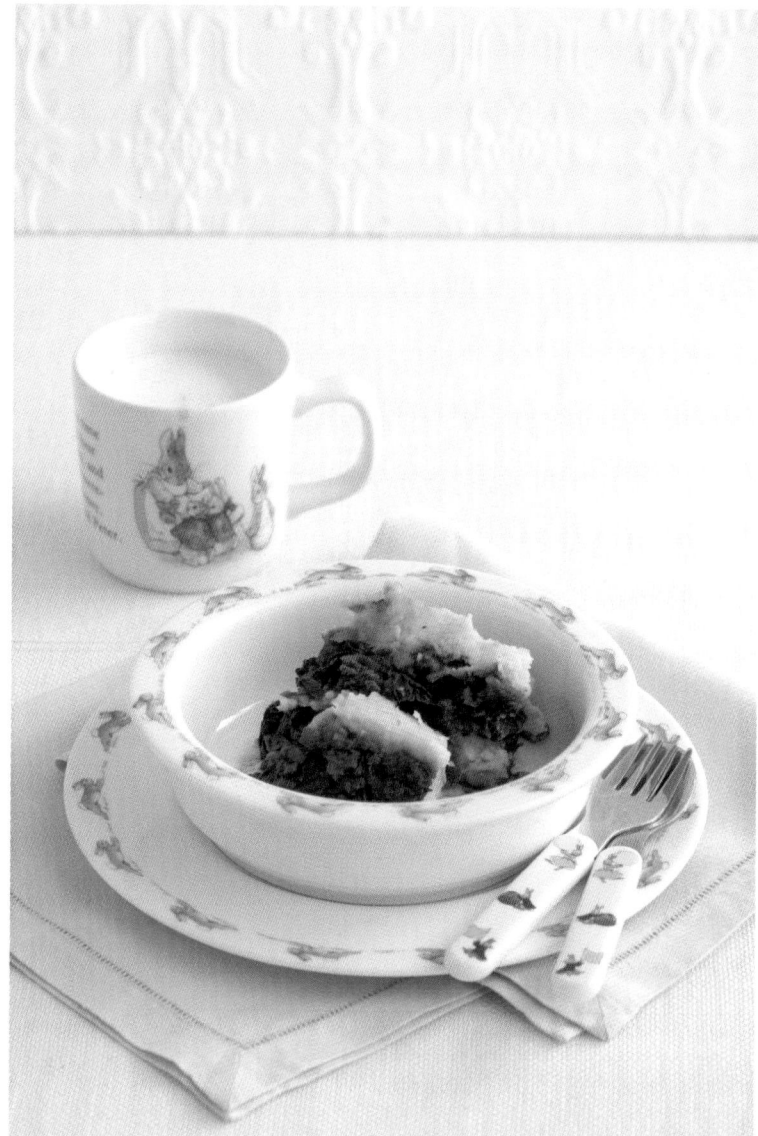

1 Heat oil in large saucepan; cook onion and garlic, stirring, until onion softens. Add beef, carrot, capsicum and mushrooms; cook, stirring, until beef changes colour.

2 Add paste, wine and undrained tomatoes; bring to a boil. Reduce heat; simmer, uncovered, about 30 minutes or until sauce thickens. Stir spinach into bolognese sauce.

3 Meanwhile, preheat oven to moderate.

4 Boil, steam or microwave potatoes until tender; drain. Mash potatoes in large bowl with butter, garlic and egg until smooth.

5 Spread half of the potato mixture over base and sides of 1.5-litre (6 cup) pie dish; spread bolognese sauce over potato then gently spread remaining potato mixture over bolognese sauce. Sprinkle with cheese.

6 Cook pie, uncovered, in moderate oven 30 minutes or until browned lightly.

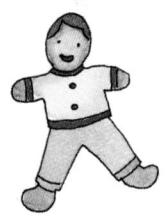

potato and bacon soup

PREPARATION TIME **15 MINUTES**
COOKING TIME **25 MINUTES** SERVES **4**

40g butter

1 medium brown onion (150g), chopped finely

1 clove garlic, crushed

4 bacon rashers (280g), rind removed, chopped coarsely

¼ cup (35g) plain flour

2 cups (500ml) chicken stock

2 cups (500ml) milk

3 medium potatoes (600g), chopped coarsely

½ cup (125ml) cream

2 tablespoons finely chopped fresh chives

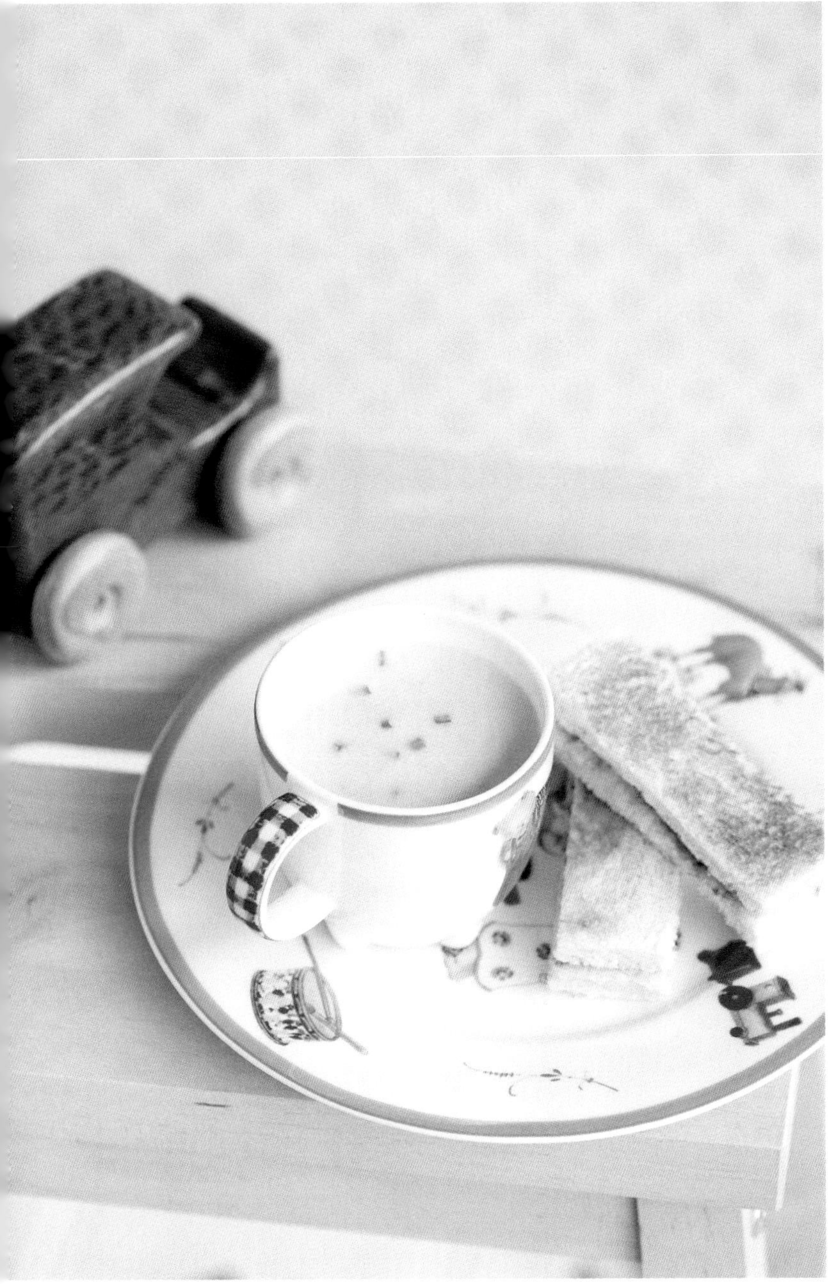

1 Heat butter in large saucepan; cook onion, garlic and bacon, stirring, until onion softens.

2 Add flour; cook, stirring, until mixture thickens and bubbles. Gradually add stock and milk; stir until mixture boils and thickens.

3 Stir in potato; return to a boil. Reduce heat; simmer, covered, about 20 minutes or until potato softens. Stir in cream and chives.

TODDLER TIP Purée toddler portion of soup before adding chives.

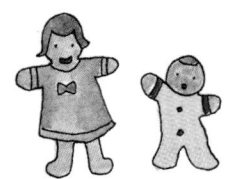

honey and soy drumsticks with easy fried rice

PREPARATION TIME **15 MINUTES (PLUS STANDING TIME)** COOKING TIME **40 MINUTES** SERVES **4**

You need to cook 1½ cups (300g) white long-grain rice the day before for this recipe.

⅓ cup (80ml) soy sauce

¼ cup (90g) honey

8 chicken drumsticks (1.2kg)

2 teaspoons vegetable oil

2 eggs, beaten lightly

4 bacon rashers (280g), rind removed, chopped coarsely

1 medium brown onion (150g), chopped finely

1 trimmed celery stick (100g), chopped finely

3 cups (600g) cooked white long-grain rice

½ cup (80g) frozen corn kernels, thawed

½ cup (60g) frozen peas, thawed

2 tablespoons soy sauce, extra

2 green onions, chopped finely

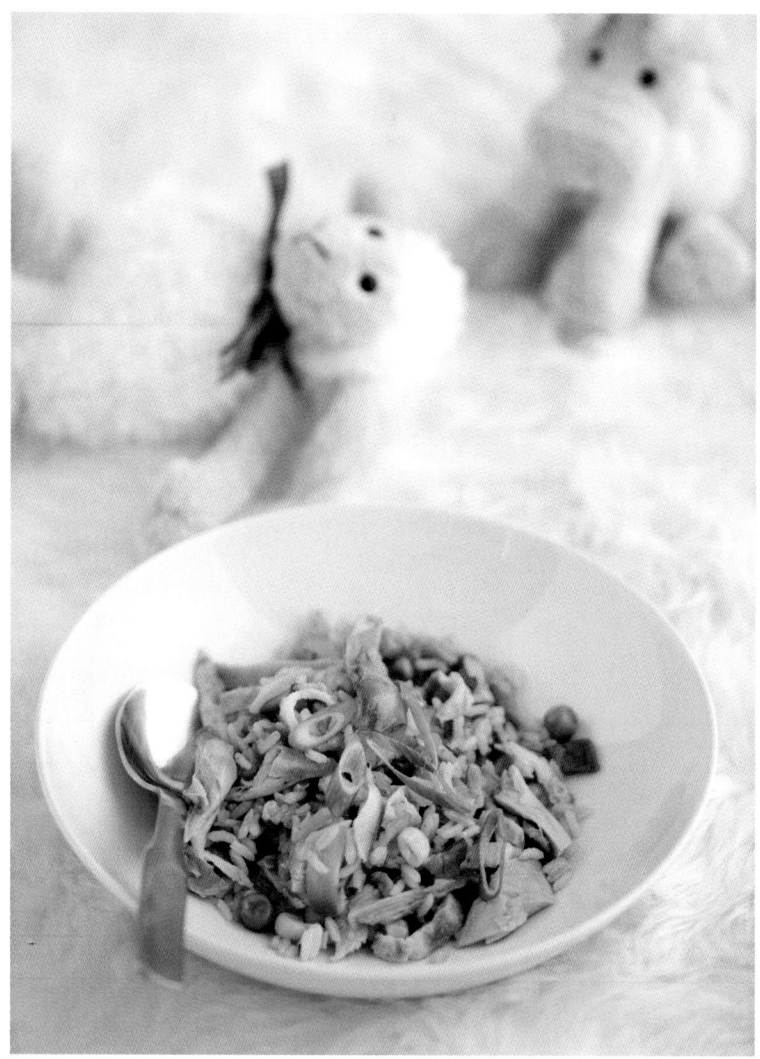

1 Combine soy and honey in large bowl, add chicken; turn chicken to coat in marinade. Cover; refrigerate 3 hours or overnight.

2 Preheat oven to moderate.

3 Place undrained chicken, in single layer, in large shallow baking dish; cook, uncovered, in moderate oven about 40 minutes or until cooked through, turning occasionally.

4 Meanwhile, heat ½ teaspoon of the oil in wok; cook half of the egg mixture over medium heat, swirling wok to make a thin omelette. Transfer to board; when cool enough to handle, roll into cigar shape, slice thinly. Repeat with another ½ teaspoon of the oil and remaining egg.

5 Heat remaining oil in same wok; stir-fry bacon, brown onion and celery until onion softens. Add rice, corn, peas and extra soy; stir-fry until heated through.

6 Sprinkle green onion over fried rice before serving with chicken.

TODDLER TIP Remove skin from chicken and cut the meat off the bone for your toddler, if desired.

crumbed fish with honey and soy baked vegetables

PREPARATION TIME 20 MINUTES (PLUS REFRIGERATION TIME) COOKING TIME 30 MINUTES SERVES 4

500g firm white fish fillets

¼ cup (35g) plain flour

2 eggs, beaten lightly

1 tablespoon finely chopped
   fresh flat-leaf parsley

1½ cups (110g) stale breadcrumbs

400g small potatoes, quartered

400g pumpkin, chopped coarsely

2 medium carrots (240g),
   chopped coarsely

2 tablespoons honey

1 tablespoon soy sauce

1 tablespoon vegetable oil

olive oil, for shallow-frying

1 Preheat oven to hot.
2 Halve fish fillets lengthways.
   Coat fish pieces, one at
   a time, in flour, then egg,
   then in combined parsley
   and breadcrumbs. Place in
   single layer on tray, cover;
   refrigerate 15 minutes.
3 Meanwhile, boil, steam or
   microwave potato, pumpkin
   and carrot, separately, until
   just tender; drain.
4 Combine vegetables with
   honey, soy and vegetable oil
   in large shallow baking dish;
   roast, uncovered, in hot oven
   about 30 minutes or until
   vegetables are browned.
5 Heat olive oil in large deep
   frying pan; shallow-fry fish,
   in batches, until browned
   lightly and cooked through.
   Drain on absorbent paper.
6 Serve fish with vegetables.

TODDLER TIP Save a small
piece of uncrumbed fish for
toddler, cooking it in the oven,
wrapped in oiled foil, for
about the last 5 minutes of
vegetable roasting time. Cut
into bite-size pieces, checking
there are no bones, and serve
with a few tablespoons of the
vegetables, mashed.

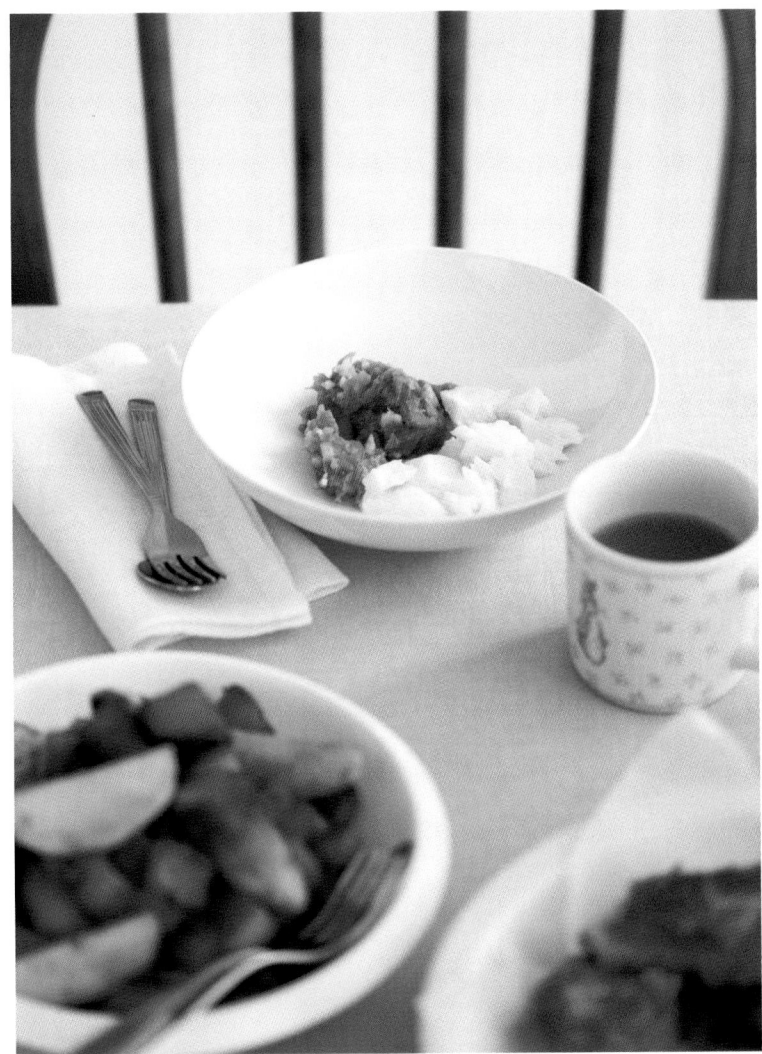

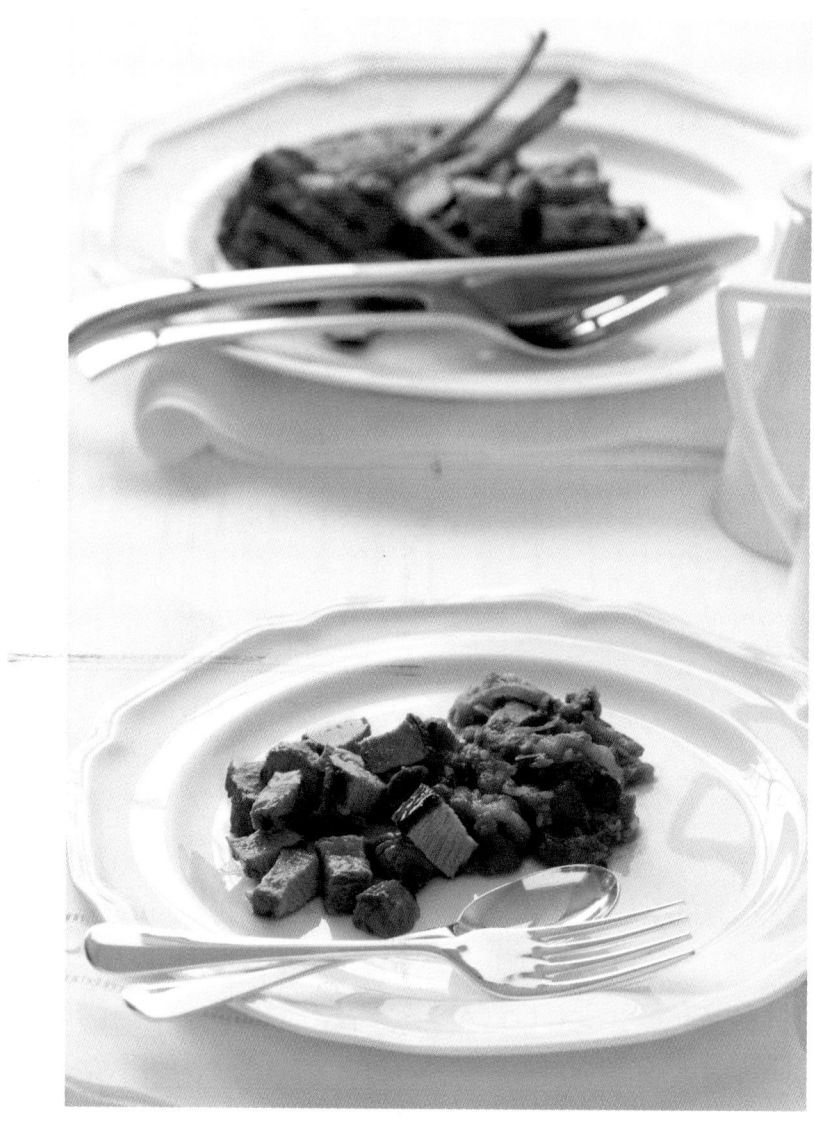

lamb cutlets with ratatouille

PREPARATION TIME 15 MINUTES   COOKING TIME 35 MINUTES   SERVES 4

2 tablespoons olive oil

1 medium red onion (170g), sliced thinly

1 large red capsicum (350g), chopped coarsely

3 large zucchini (450g), sliced thickly

5 baby eggplants (300g), sliced thickly

400g can diced tomatoes

1 tablespoon tomato paste

2 cloves garlic, crushed

12 french-trimmed lamb cutlets (900g)

1 Heat oil in large saucepan; cook onion, capsicum, zucchini and eggplant, stirring, 5 minutes. Add undrained tomatoes and paste; bring to a boil. Reduce heat; simmer, covered, about 20 minutes or until vegetables have softened. Stir in garlic.

2 Meanwhile, cook cutlets on heated oiled grill plate (or grill or barbecue) until cooked as desired. Serve with ratatouille.

TODDLER TIP Cut the meat from one cutlet; trim it of all fat then cut into bite-size pieces and serve with a few tablespoons of mashed ratatouille.

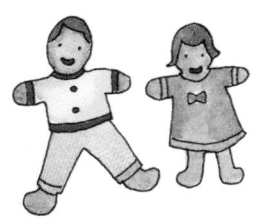

fettuccine with tuna, tomato and eggplant

PREPARATION TIME **10 MINUTES**   COOKING TIME **15 MINUTES**   SERVES **4**

375g tri-colour fettuccine

1 tablespoon finely grated lemon rind

½ cup coarsely chopped fresh flat-leaf parsley

1 tablespoon olive oil

6 large egg tomatoes (540g), chopped coarsely

280g jar char-grilled eggplant, drained, chopped coarsely

425g can tuna in springwater, drained, flaked

1 Cook pasta in large saucepan of boiling water, uncovered, until just tender; drain. Combine in large bowl with rind, parsley and oil.

2 Meanwhile, cook tomato, uncovered, in oiled large frying pan until just softened. Add eggplant and tuna; cook, uncovered, until heated through.

3 Add tomato mixture to pasta mixture; toss gently to combine.

TODDLER TIP Cut the fettuccine into lengths your toddler can manage easily.

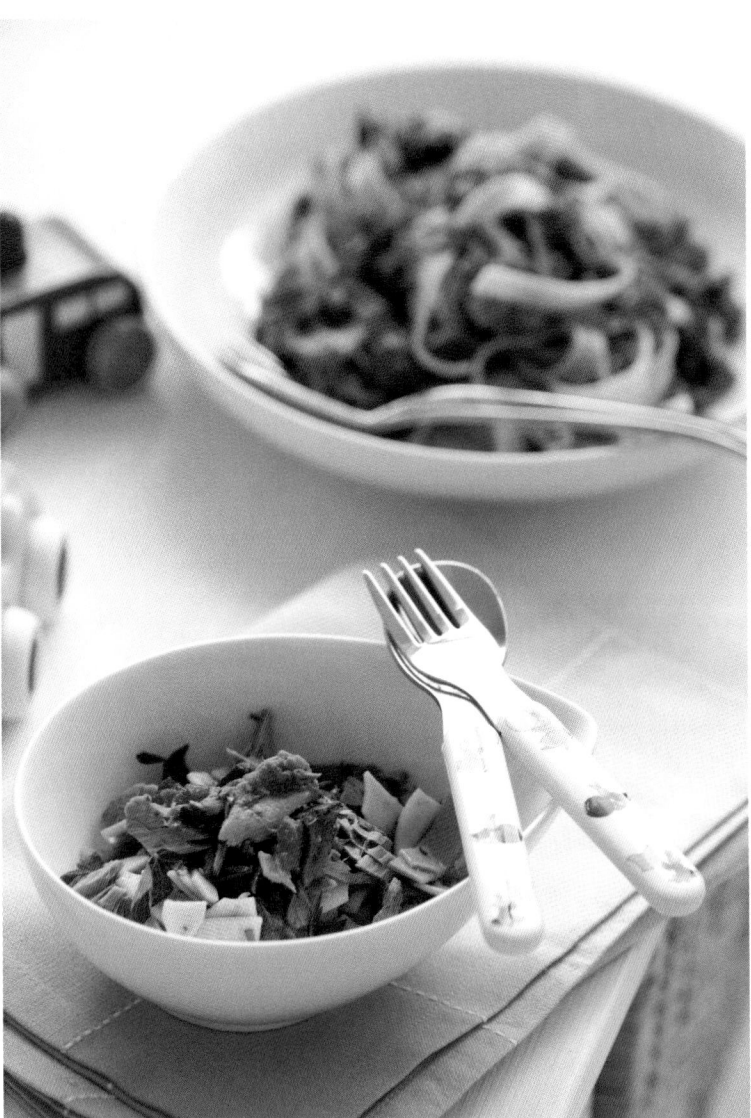

73

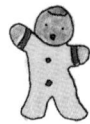

fish and salad burgers

PREPARATION TIME 30 MINUTES
(PLUS REFRIGERATION TIME)
COOKING TIME 15 MINUTES SERVES 4

1 large potato (300g),
    chopped coarsely

1 tablespoon vegetable oil

1 medium brown onion (150g),
    chopped finely

1 clove garlic, crushed

415g can pink salmon, drained

2 teaspoons finely grated
    lemon rind

1 tablespoon finely chopped
    fresh chives

1 egg

¼ cup (35g) plain flour

1 egg, beaten lightly, extra

1 cup (70g) stale breadcrumbs

vegetable oil, extra, for
    shallow-frying

4 hot dog rolls

¼ cup (75g) tartare sauce

1 medium carrot (120g),
    grated coarsely

½ butter lettuce (100g),
    shredded coarsely

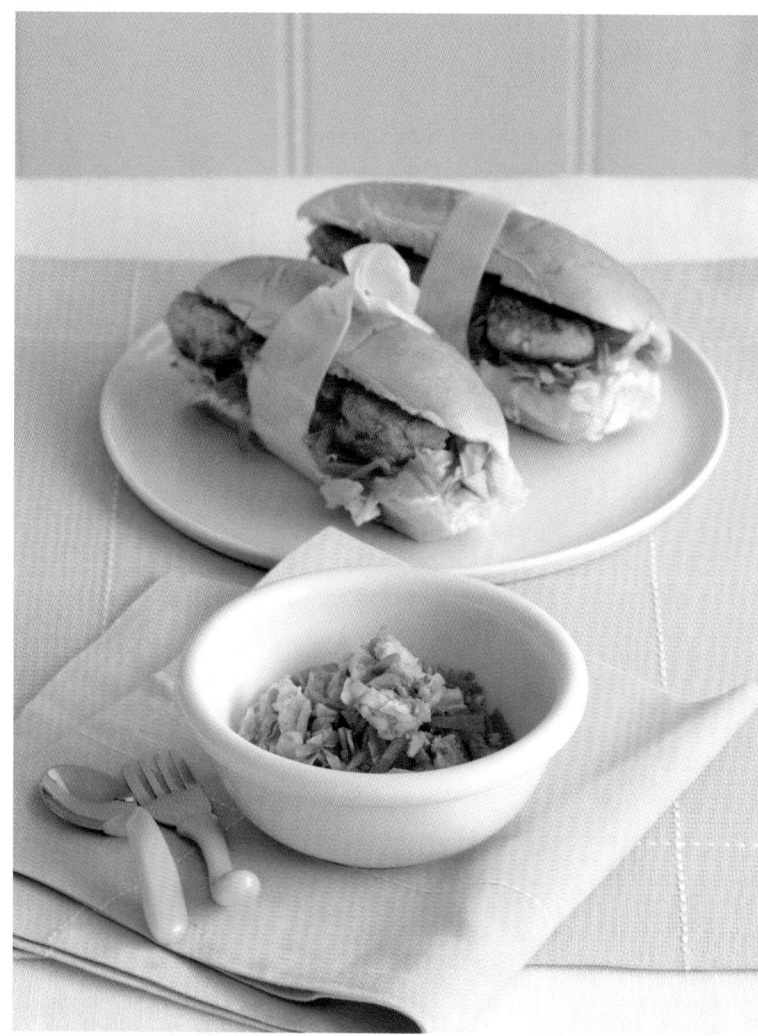

1 Boil, steam or microwave potato until tender; drain. Mash in medium bowl.
2 Meanwhile, heat oil in medium frying pan, cook onion and garlic, stirring, until onion softens.
3 Discard any bones from salmon; flake into bowl with potato. Add onion mixture, rind, chives and egg; use hand to combine. Roll rounded tablespoons of burger mixture into balls; flatten into slightly oval-shaped burgers (you will have 16 burgers).
4 Coat burgers with flour; shake away excess. Dip into extra egg then breadcrumbs. Cover; refrigerate 1 hour.
5 Heat oil in large frying pan; shallow-fry burgers, in batches, until cooked through. Drain on absorbent paper.
6 Halve rolls; spread sauce over cut sides, sandwich burgers, carrot and lettuce between roll halves.

TODDLER TIP Give your toddler one mashed or chopped fish burger with a little of the carrot and lettuce.

chicken schnitzel burgers

PREPARATION TIME 35 MINUTES (PLUS REFRIGERATION TIME)   COOKING TIME 35 MINUTES   SERVES 4

4 single chicken breast fillets (680g)

¼ cup (35g) plain flour

1 egg

1 tablespoon milk

1 cup (70g) stale breadcrumbs

¼ cup (60ml) olive oil

3 medium red onions (510g), sliced thinly

1 loaf turkish bread (430g), cut into four pieces

⅓ iceberg lettuce (200g), shredded coarsely

CAPSICUM AND CAPER MAYONNAISE

¼ cup (75g) mayonnaise

⅓ cup (65g) char-grilled red capsicum, chopped finely

1 tablespoon drained capers, rinsed, chopped coarsely

1 Using meat mallet, gently pound fillets between pieces of plastic wrap until 1cm thick. Toss chicken in flour; shake away excess. Dip into combined egg and milk then breadcrumbs. Cover; refrigerate 1 hour.

2 Meanwhile, combine ingredients for capsicum and caper mayonnaise in small bowl. Cover; refrigerate until required.

3 Heat 1 tablespoon of the oil in large frying pan; cook onion, uncovered, stirring occasionally, about 15 minutes or until caramelised. Transfer to small bowl; cover to keep warm.

4 Heat remaining oil in same cleaned frying pan; cook chicken, in batches, until cooked through. Drain on absorbent paper; cover to keep warm.

5 Meanwhile, split bread pieces in half; toast cut sides of bread. Sandwich chicken, onion, mayonnaise and lettuce between bread halves.

TODDLER TIP Cut part of one of the schnitzels into finger-size pieces and serve with tomato sauce instead of the capsicum and caper mayonnaise.

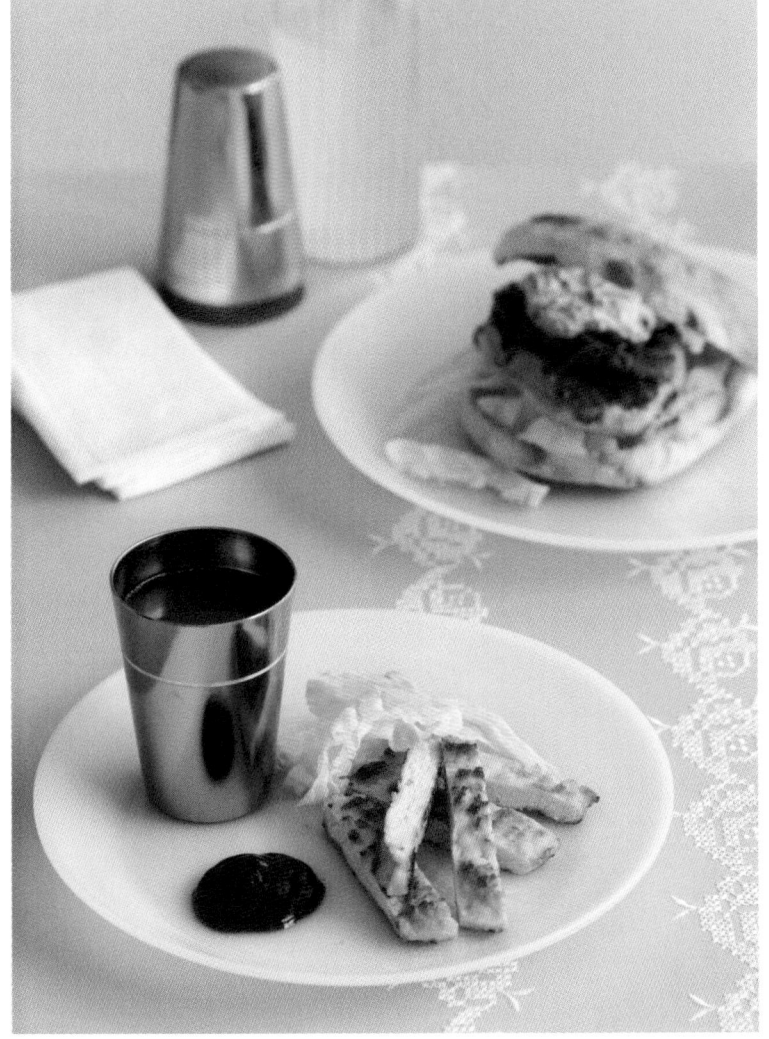

apple and sultana strudel with custard

PREPARATION TIME **20 MINUTES** COOKING TIME **20 MINUTES** SERVES **4**

2 tablespoons raw sugar

1 teaspoon ground cinnamon

2 sheets ready-rolled puff
  pastry, thawed

425g can pie apple

½ cup (80g) sultanas

1 egg, beaten lightly

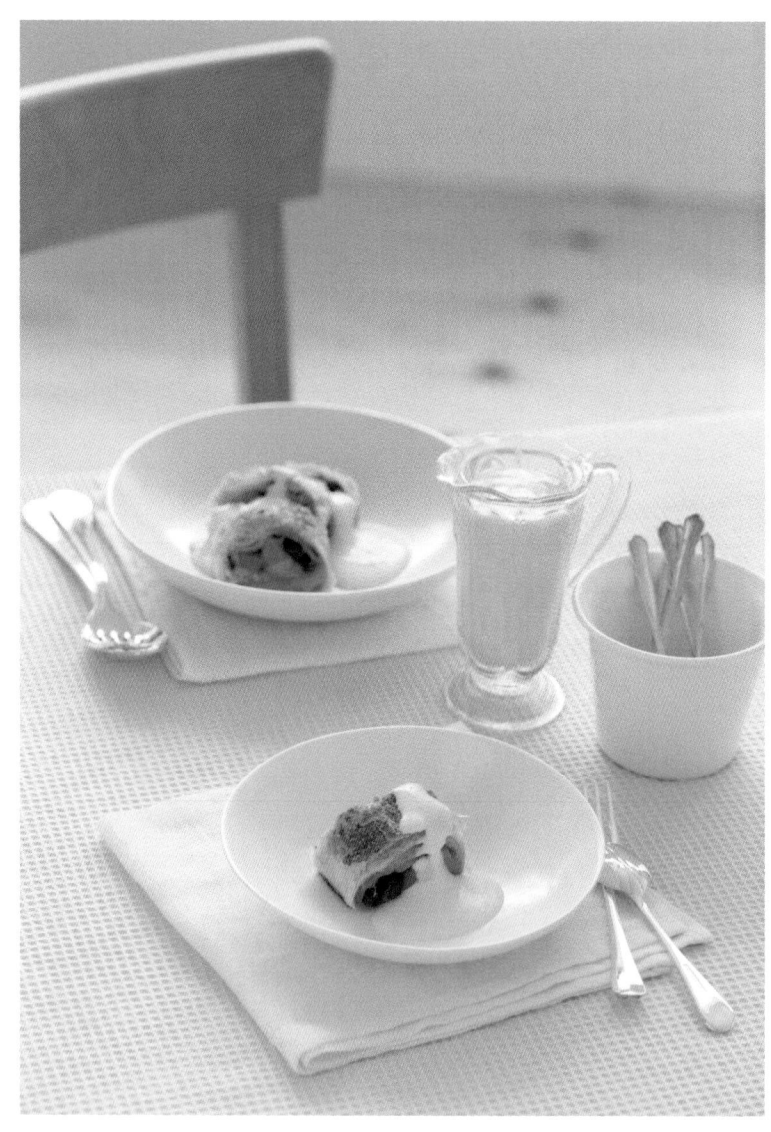

1 Preheat oven to moderately
   hot. Grease two oven trays.

2 Combine sugar and
   cinnamon in small bowl.

3 Sprinkle 2 teaspoons of
   the sugar mixture over one
   pastry sheet. Place half of
   the pie apple on one half of
   pastry sheet; sprinkle with
   half of the sultanas. Roll
   pastry carefully to enclose
   filling. Repeat process with
   another 2 teaspoons of the
   sugar mixture and remaining
   pastry sheet, pie apple
   and sultanas.

4 Place strudels, seam-side
   down, on prepared trays;
   brush with egg, sprinkle
   each with remaining sugar
   mixture. Bake strudels,
   uncovered, in moderately hot
   oven about 20 minutes or
   until browned lightly. Stand
   10 minutes before slicing.

TODDLER TIP Serve toddler a
small piece of warm strudel,
with custard or vanilla ice-cream.

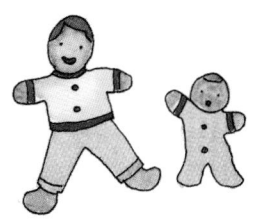

frozen yogurt and raspberry swirl

PREPARATION TIME 15 MINUTES (PLUS FREEZING TIME) COOKING TIME 5 MINUTES SERVES 4

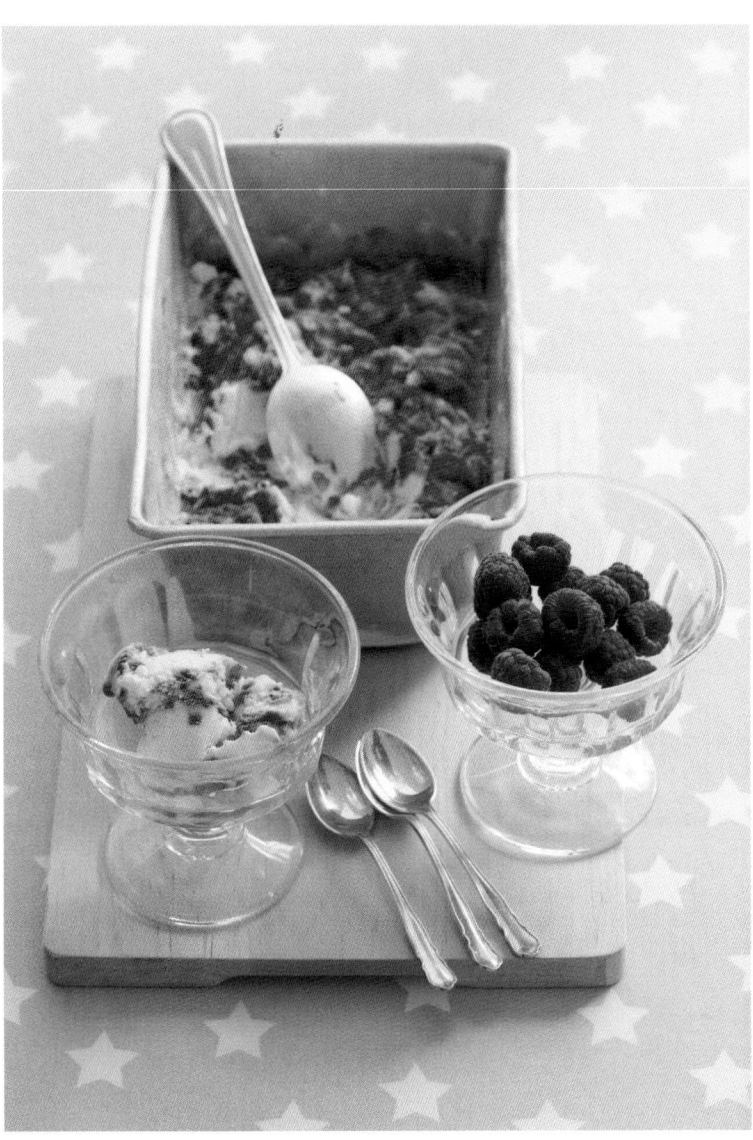

²/₃ cup (150g) caster sugar
⅓ cup (80ml) water
1 teaspoon gelatine
120g frozen raspberries
500g thick greek-style yogurt

1 Combine sugar and the water in small saucepan, stir over low heat until sugar dissolves; cool 5 minutes. Sprinkle gelatine over syrup; stir until gelatine dissolves.
2 Push raspberries through fine sieve over small bowl; discard seeds.
3 Combine gelatine mixture and yogurt in medium bowl; pour into 14cm x 21cm loaf pan. Cover; freeze about 4 hours or until almost firm.
4 Uncover, scrape yogurt from bottom and sides of pan with fork; swirl raspberry through yogurt. Cover; freeze until ready to serve. Serve with fresh raspberries, if desired.

TODDLER TIP Break up a few tablespoons of the frozen yogurt and raspberry swirl with a fork in toddler's bowl.

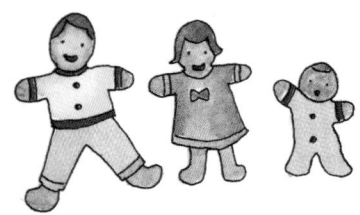

apple and
berry crumble

PREPARATION TIME 15 MINUTES
COOKING TIME 25 MINUTES SERVES 6

800g can pie apple

2 cups (300g) frozen
   mixed berries

1 tablespoon white sugar

½ cup (125ml) water

1 cup (120g) toasted muesli

2 tablespoons plain flour

1 tablespoon brown sugar

50g butter

½ cup (20g) corn flakes

1 Preheat oven to moderate.

2 Combine pie apple, berries,
   white sugar and the water in
   medium saucepan; bring to
   a boil. Reduce heat; simmer,
   stirring, until mixture is
   combined. Remove from heat.

3 Meanwhile, combine muesli,
   flour and brown sugar in
   medium bowl. Use fingertips to
   rub in butter; stir in cornflakes.

4 Place apple mixture in
   2-litre (8 cup) ovenproof dish;
   sprinkle with muesli mixture.
   Bake, uncovered, in moderate
   oven about 20 minutes or
   until browned lightly.

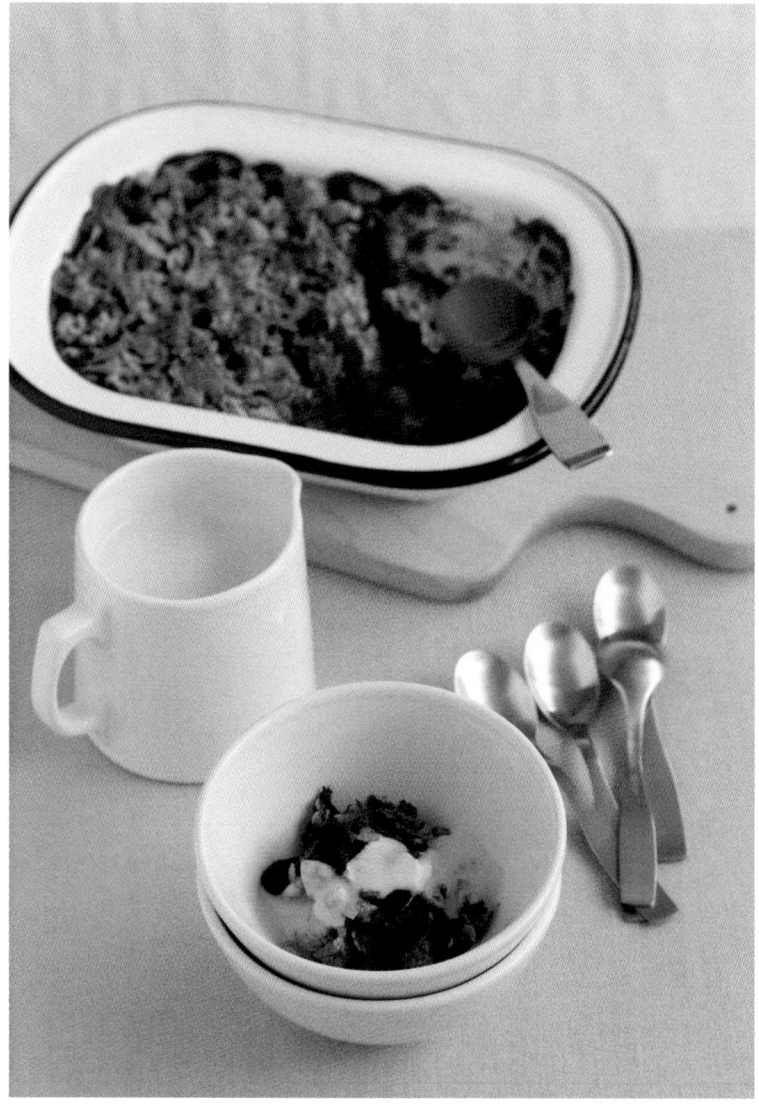

TODDLER TIPS You can
substitute pear for the apple,
if you like, or even a single
berry variety. Fresh or frozen
berries can be used. Give your
toddler a few tablespoons
of the warm crumble topped
with custard.

Make sure you use a muesli
that does not contain large
chunks of nuts or seeds.

creamed rice with dried fruit compote

PREPARATION TIME **20 MINUTES (PLUS STANDING TIME)** COOKING TIME **1 HOUR 5 MINUTES** SERVES **4**

1 litre (4 cups) milk

⅓ cup (75g) caster sugar

10cm strip lemon rind

⅓ cup (65g) white medium-grain rice

2 teaspoons cornflour

1 tablespoon water

2 egg yolks

½ teaspoon vanilla extract

DRIED FRUIT COMPOTE

½ cup (75g) coarsely chopped dried pear

½ cup (45g) coarsely chopped dried apple

½ cup (85g) coarsely chopped seeded prunes

2 cups (500ml) water

2 tablespoons honey

1 Combine milk in medium saucepan with sugar and rind; bring to a boil, stirring occasionally. Gradually stir in rice, reduce heat; simmer, covered, about 40 minutes or until rice is tender, stirring occasionally. Discard rind.

2 Meanwhile, make dried fruit compote.

3 Blend cornflour with the water in small bowl; stir in egg yolks. Stir in a heaped tablespoon of the hot creamed rice then pour egg mixture into creamed rice. Stir over medium heat until mixture boils and thickens. Stir in extract; remove from heat. Stand 15 minutes before serving with compote.

dried fruit compote Place ingredients in medium saucepan; bring to a boil. Reduce heat; simmer, uncovered, 15 minutes. Remove from heat.

TODDLER TIP Purée a few tablespoons of the compote and stir it through a small amount of the creamed rice.

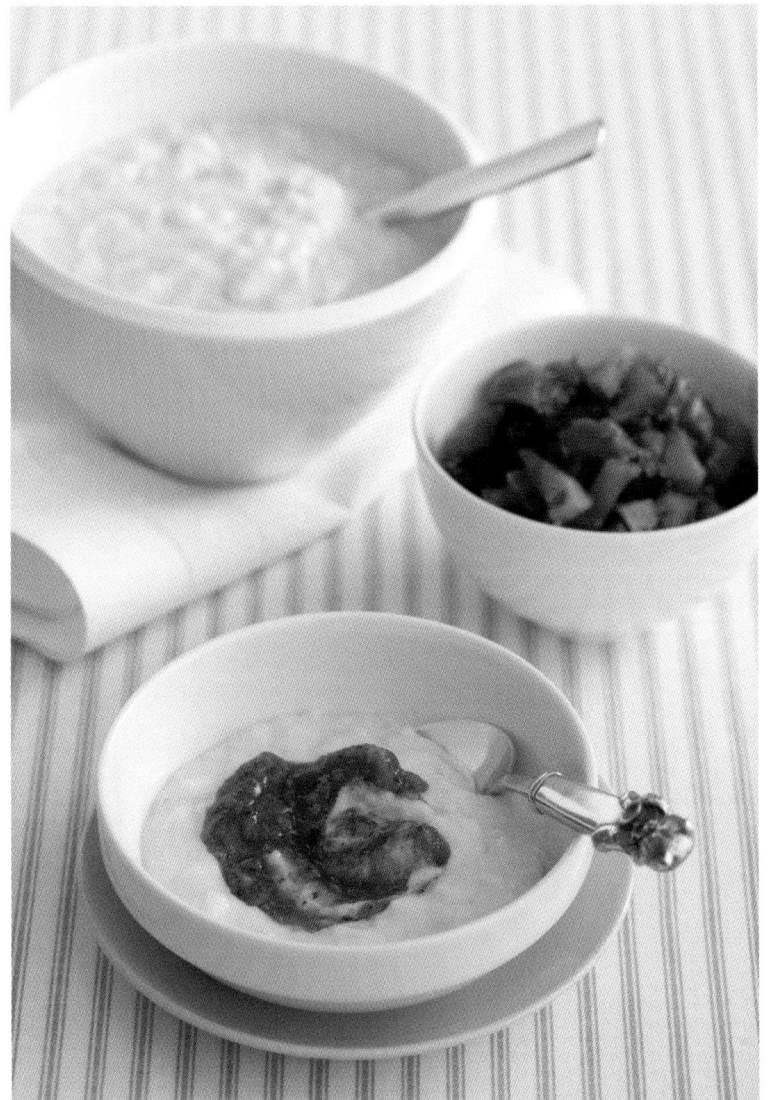

muesli slice

PREPARATION TIME **15 MINUTES**

COOKING TIME **20 MINUTES** MAKES **30**

125g butter

⅓ cup (75g) firmly packed
   brown sugar

2 tablespoons honey

1 cup (90g) rolled oats

½ cup (45g) desiccated coconut

½ cup (80g) finely chopped
   dried apricots

½ cup (75g) finely chopped
   dried apples

½ cup (80g) sultanas

½ cup (75g) self-raising flour

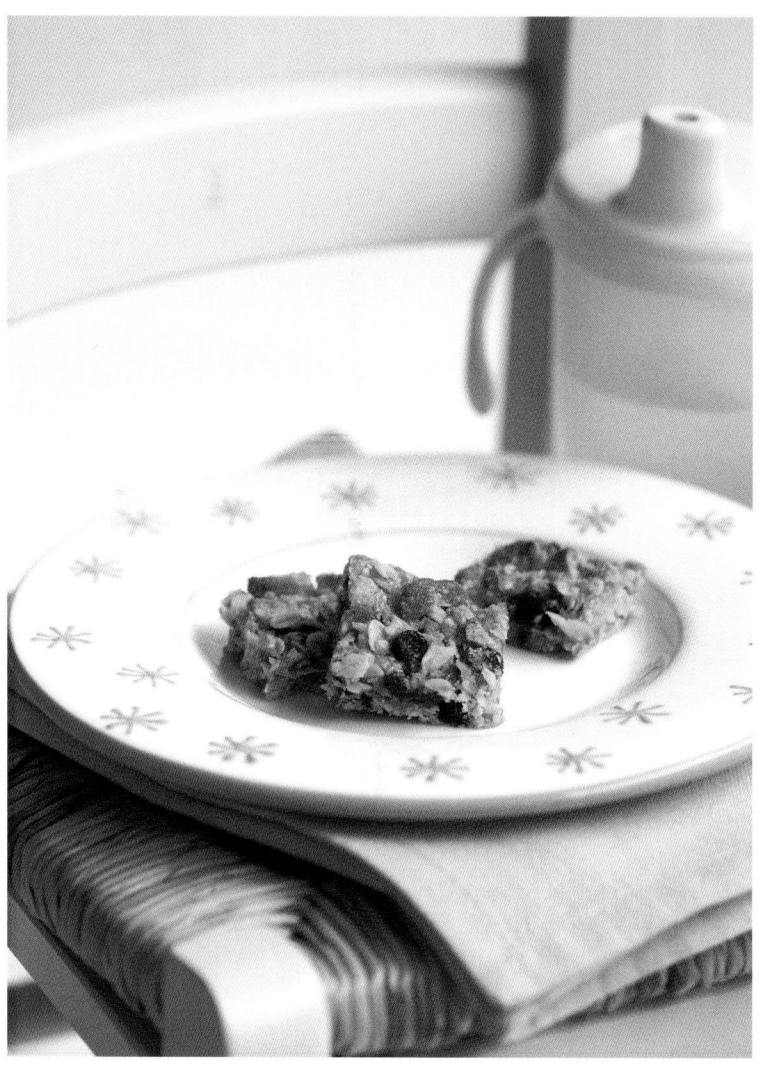

1 Preheat oven to moderate.
   Grease and line 20cm x 30cm
   lamington pan.

2 Combine butter, sugar and
   honey in large saucepan; stir
   over medium heat, without
   boiling, until sugar dissolves.
   Remove from heat; stir in
   remaining ingredients.

3 Press mixture into prepared
   pan. Bake, uncovered,
   in moderate oven about
   20 minutes or until golden
   brown. Cool in pan; cut
   into squares to serve.

TODDLER TIP Chop toddler
pieces finely then stir through
soft vanilla ice-cream or yogurt.

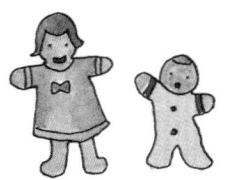

abc mini muffins (apple, banana, chocolate)

PREPARATION TIME **15 MINUTES** COOKING TIME **15 MINUTES** MAKES **24**

¾ cup (110g) self-raising flour

⅓ cup (75g) firmly packed brown sugar

¼ cup (20g) rolled oats

1 egg

¼ cup (60ml) milk

¼ cup (60ml) apple juice

¼ cup (60ml) vegetable oil

½ medium ripe banana (100g), chopped finely

100g dark eating chocolate, grated finely

1 Preheat oven to moderate. Line two 12-hole (1 tablespoon/20ml) mini muffin pans with patty-pan cases.

2 Combine flour, sugar and oats in medium bowl. Stir in combined egg, milk, juice and oil. Add banana and half of the chocolate; stir gently to just combine.

3 Divide mixture among prepared holes of pans. Bake, uncovered, in moderate oven about 15 minutes. Stand muffins in pans 5 minutes; turn onto wire rack, sprinkle with remaining chocolate.

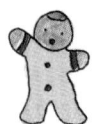

mini pineapple and carrot cakes

PREPARATION TIME **10 MINUTES**   COOKING TIME **15 MINUTES**   MAKES **24**

⅓ cup (50g) plain flour

½ cup (75g) self-raising flour

½ teaspoon bicarbonate of soda

¼ cup (55g) caster sugar

½ teaspoon ground cinnamon

225g can crushed pineapple, drained

⅔ cup (160g) firmly packed finely grated carrot

⅓ cup (80ml) vegetable oil

1 egg, beaten lightly

CREAM CHEESE ICING

125g cream cheese, softened

1 tablespoon icing sugar mixture

1 teaspoon lemon juice

2 teaspoons milk

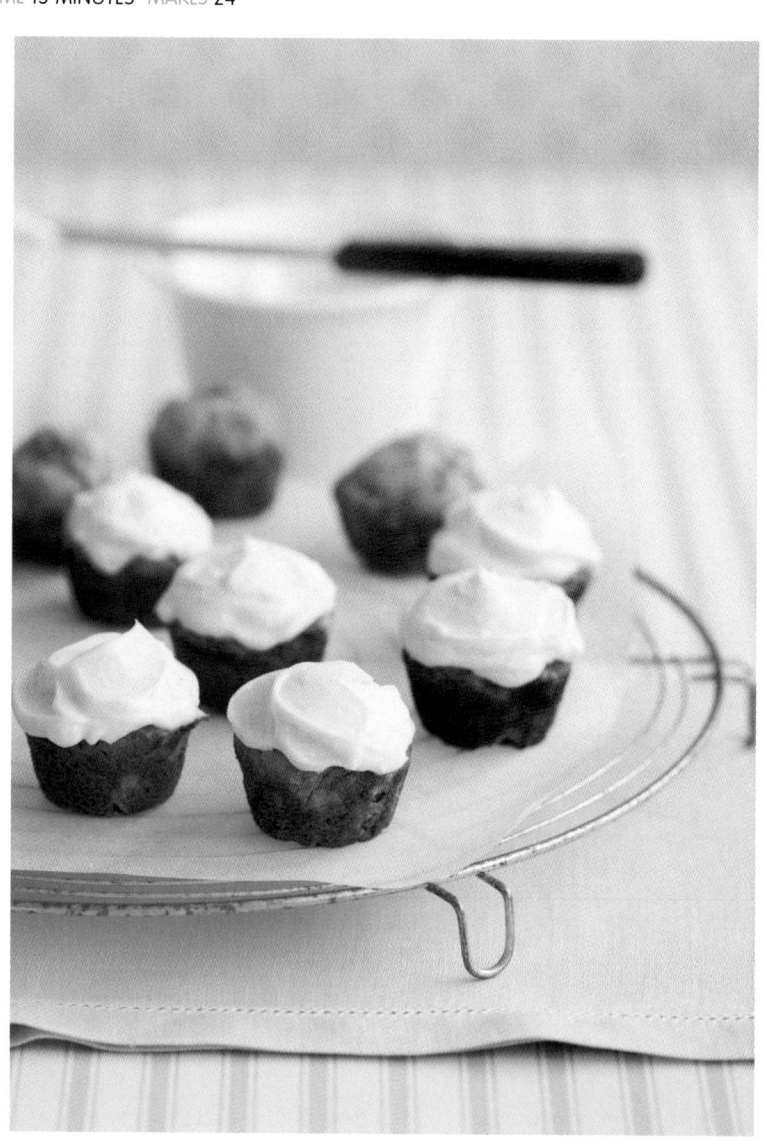

1 Preheat oven to moderate. Grease two 12-hole (1 tablespoon/20ml) mini muffin pans.

2 Sift flours, soda, sugar and cinnamon into medium bowl. Add pineapple and carrot; stir in combined oil and egg (do not over-mix).

3 Divide mixture among prepared holes. Bake, uncovered, in moderate oven about 15 minutes. Stand muffins in pans 5 minutes; turn onto wire rack to cool.

4 Meanwhile, combine ingredients for cream cheese icing in small bowl. Spread cooled muffins with icing.

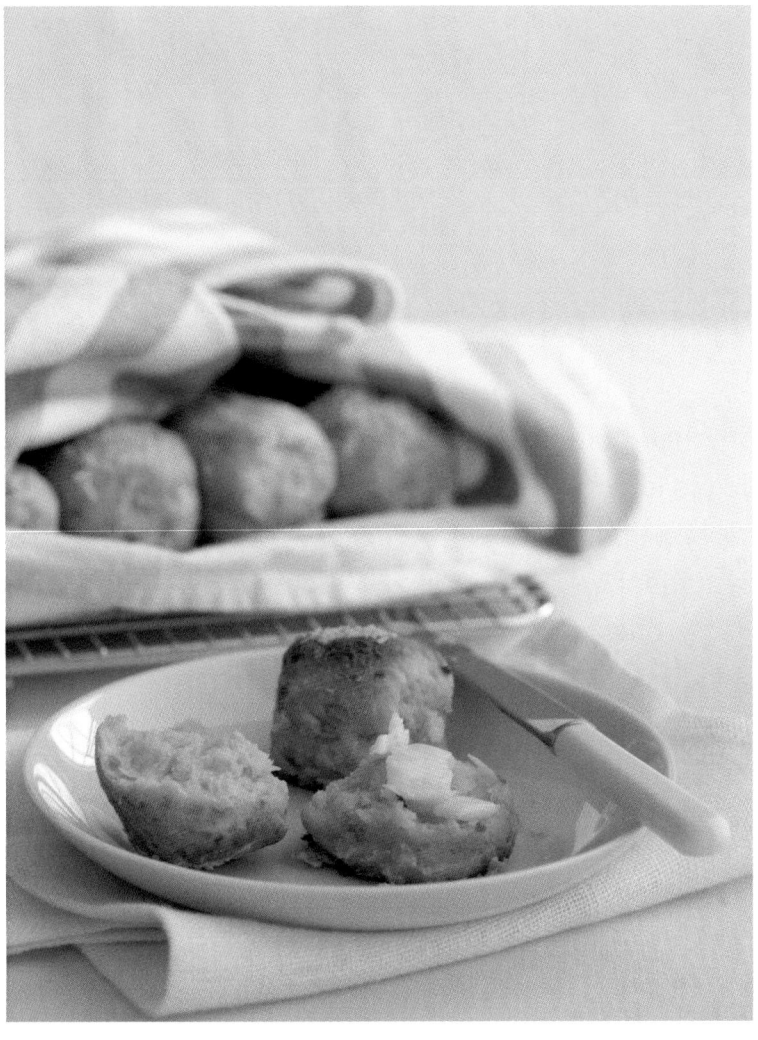

pumpkin and cheese scones

PREPARATION TIME 20 MINUTES   COOKING TIME 25 MINUTES   MAKES 16

250g pumpkin, chopped coarsely

2½ cups (375g) self-raising flour

1 tablespoon caster sugar

50g butter, chopped

¼ cup (30g) coarsely grated cheddar

¼ cup (20g) coarsely grated parmesan

½ cup (125ml) milk, approximately

¼ cup (20g) coarsely grated parmesan, extra

1   Preheat oven to very hot. Grease deep 19cm-square cake pan.

2   Boil, steam or microwave pumpkin until just tender; drain. Mash pumpkin in small bowl; cool 10 minutes.

3   Place flour and sugar in medium bowl; use fingertips to rub in butter. Stir in cheeses and pumpkin. Make well in centre of mixture; add only enough milk to mix to a soft, sticky dough. Turn dough onto lightly floured surface; knead lightly until smooth.

4   Press dough out to about 2cm in thickness; cut 16 x 4.5cm rounds from dough. Place scones, side by side and just touching, in prepared pan; sprinkle with extra cheese. Bake, uncovered, in very hot oven about 20 minutes.

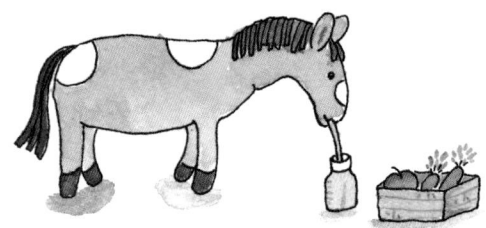

LUNCH BOXES + SNACKS

When lunching away from their homes, whether at daycare or simply on an outing, toddlers love the excitement and anticipation of peeping into their lunch box to discover what's inside. These simple and healthy ideas for lunch – or a snack – will become firm favourites with your little one.

sandwich fillings

PREPARATION TIME 10 MINUTES EACH MAKES 1

corn, zucchini and egg

Combine 2 tablespoons canned corn kernels, ½ small coarsely grated zucchini, 2 teaspoons mayonnaise and 1 mashed hard-boiled egg in small bowl. Spread egg mixture on one slice of sandwich bread; top with another slice of sandwich bread. Cut into squares or triangles.

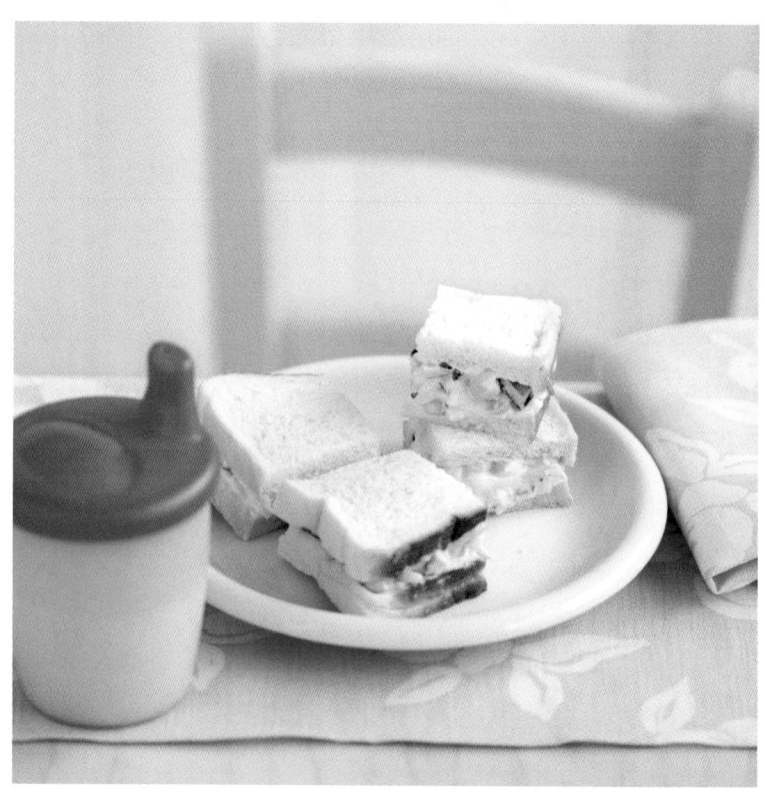

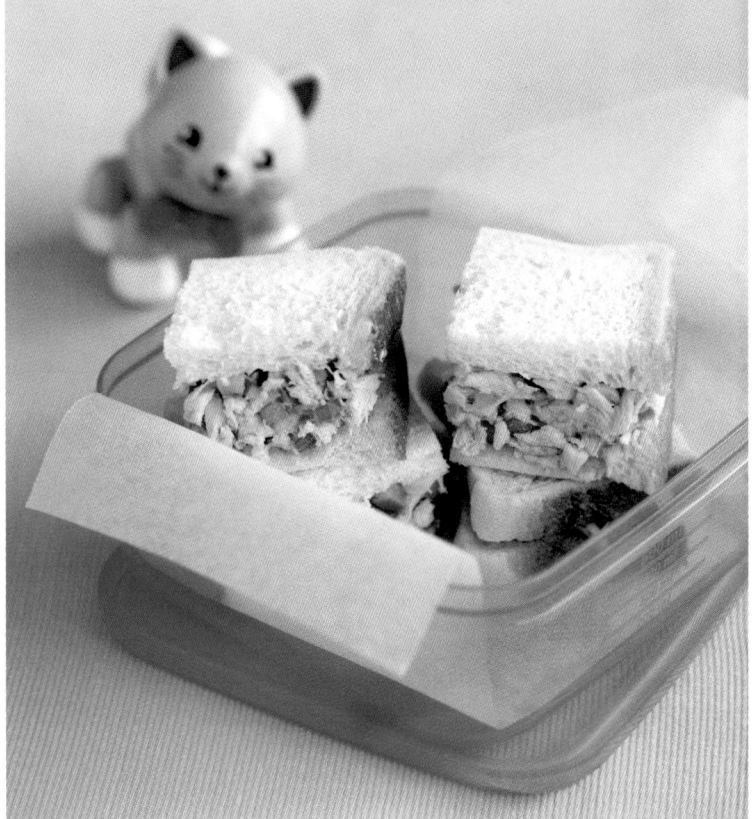

chicken, celery and avocado

Combine ⅓ cup finely shredded cooked chicken, 1 trimmed finely chopped celery stick, ¼ small avocado and 1 teaspoon lemon juice in small bowl. Spread chicken mixture on one slice of sandwich bread; top with another slice of sandwich bread. Cut into squares or triangles.

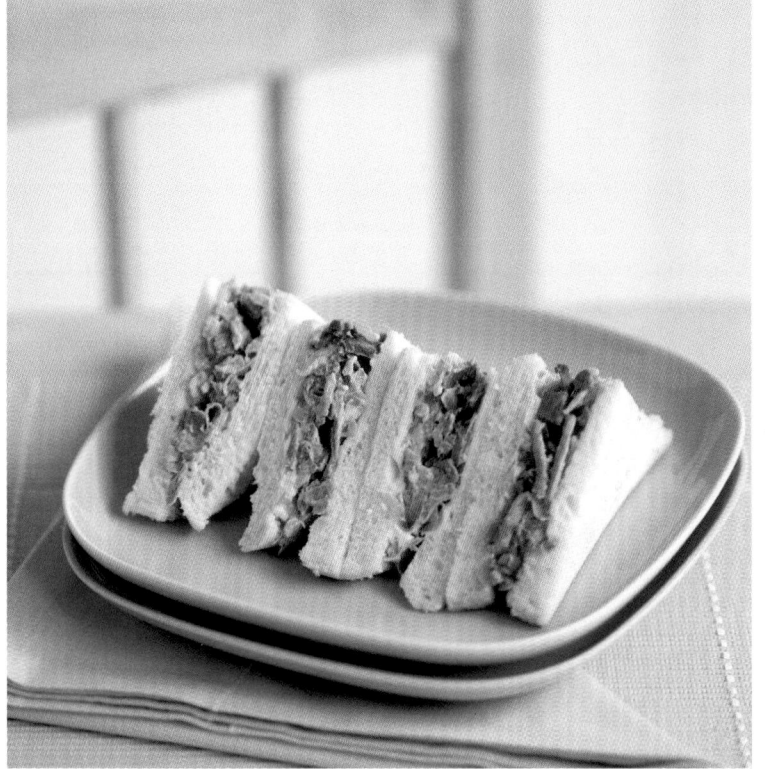

beef, cheese and carrot

Combine ½ small coarsely grated carrot, 2 tablespoons spreadable cream cheese and 2 tablespoons finely shredded iceberg lettuce in small bowl. Spread half of the carrot mixture on one slice of sandwich bread; top with ¼ cup finely chopped roast beef, remaining carrot mixture and another slice of sandwich bread. Cut into squares or triangles.

85

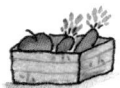

carrot dip

PREPARATION TIME 15 MINUTES

COOKING TIME 20 MINUTES MAKES 1½ CUPS

Boil, steam or microwave 5 medium coarsely chopped carrots until tender; drain. Heat 1 tablespoon olive oil in large frying pan; cook 1 crushed clove garlic and ½ teaspoon ground cumin, stirring, until fragrant. Stir in carrot and 2 teaspoons lemon juice; cook, stirring, until combined. Remove from heat; cool 10 minutes. Blend or process carrot mixture and ⅓ cup yogurt until just smooth. Serve carrot dip with grissini sticks, if desired.

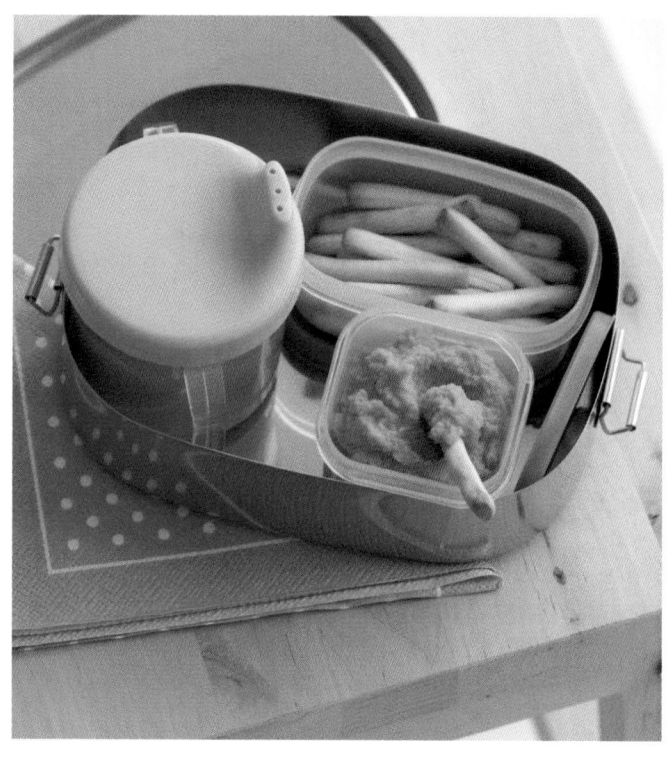

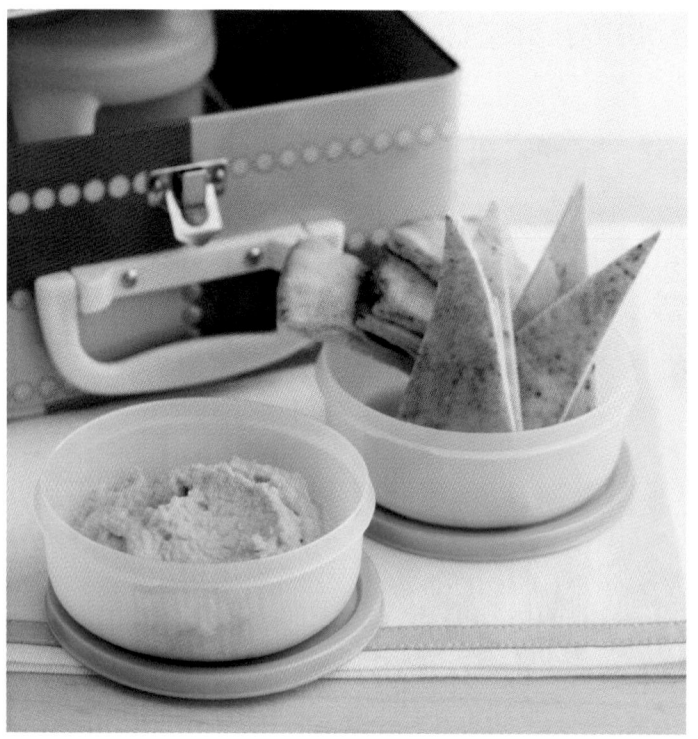

hummus

PREPARATION TIME 10 MINUTES

COOKING TIME 15 MINUTES MAKES 2 CUPS

Cook 2 x 300g cans rinsed and drained chickpeas in medium saucepan of boiling water, uncovered, about 15 minutes or until tender; drain. Cool 10 minutes. Blend or process chickpeas with 2 tablepoons olive oil, 2 teaspoons lemon juice, 1 crushed clove garlic and 1 cup yogurt until smooth. Serve hummus with pitta bread triangles, if desired.

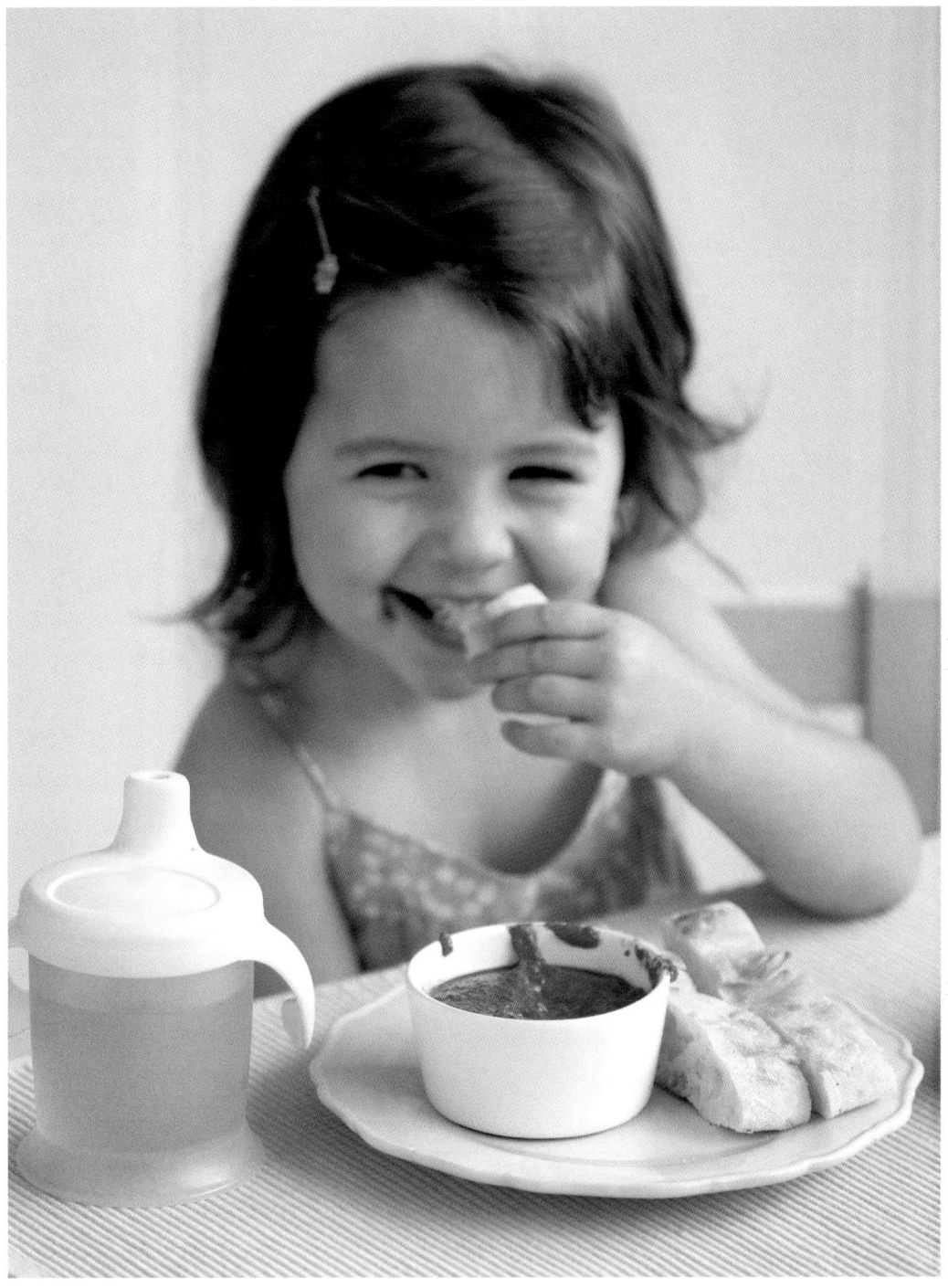

beetroot dip

PREPARATION TIME 5 MINUTES MAKES 2 CUPS

Blend or process 450g can drained baby beetroot, ½ cup thick yogurt and 1 tablespoon lemon juice until smooth.

TIP You could omit the lemon juice and replace it with water or the liquid from the beetroot, if you prefer.

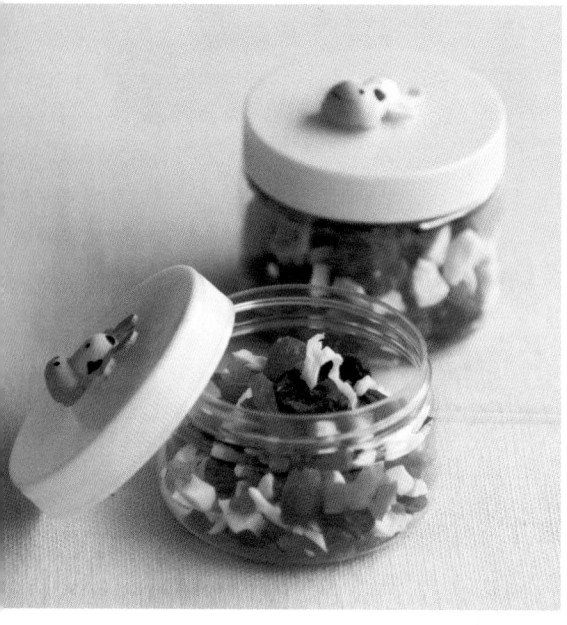

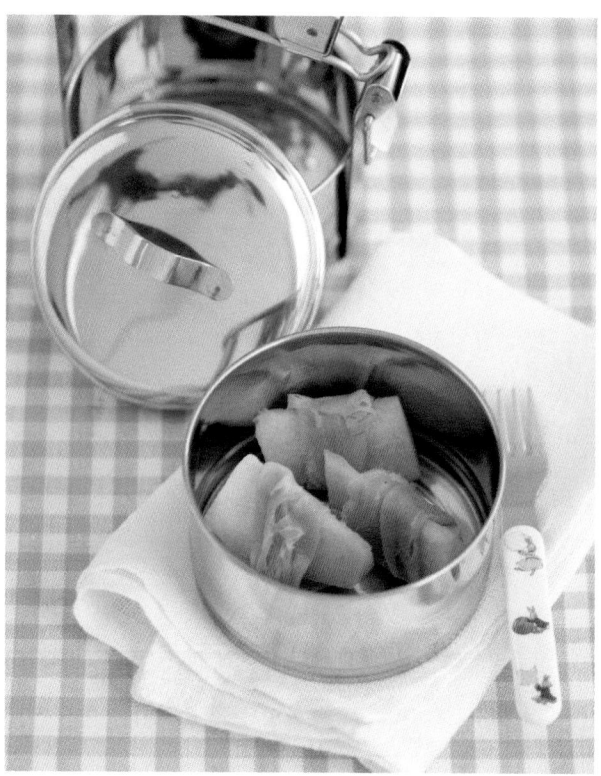

dried fruit mix

MAKES 2 CUPS

Combine ½ cup finely chopped dried pears, ½ cup finely chopped dried apricots, ⅔ cup finely chopped dried apples and ⅓ cup craisins in medium bowl.

melon and ham wraps

PREPARATION TIME 10 MINUTES

You need 160g of thinly sliced or shaved ham for this recipe.

Cut half a small peeled rockmelon lengthways into eight strips; cut each strip in half crossways. Wrap a piece of ham around each rockmelon strip.

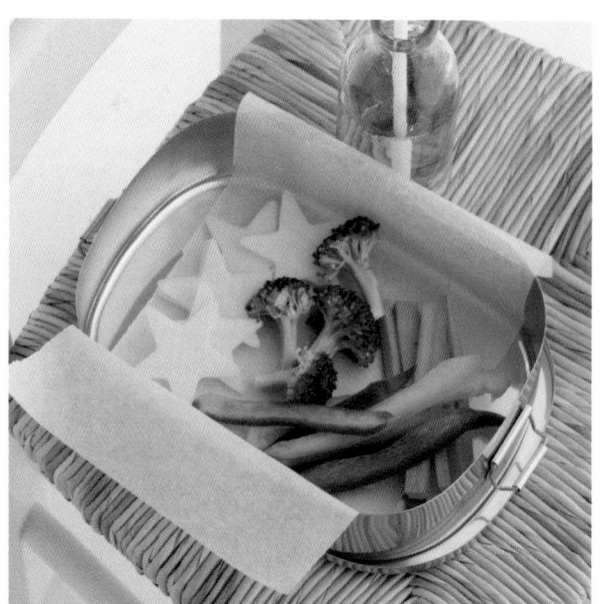

crudités

A perfect lunch box snack is assorted crudités – try using cheese slices cut into different shapes using a cookie cutter, or briefly cooked carrot sticks, broccoli florets, kumara rounds or capsicum strips.

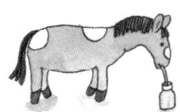

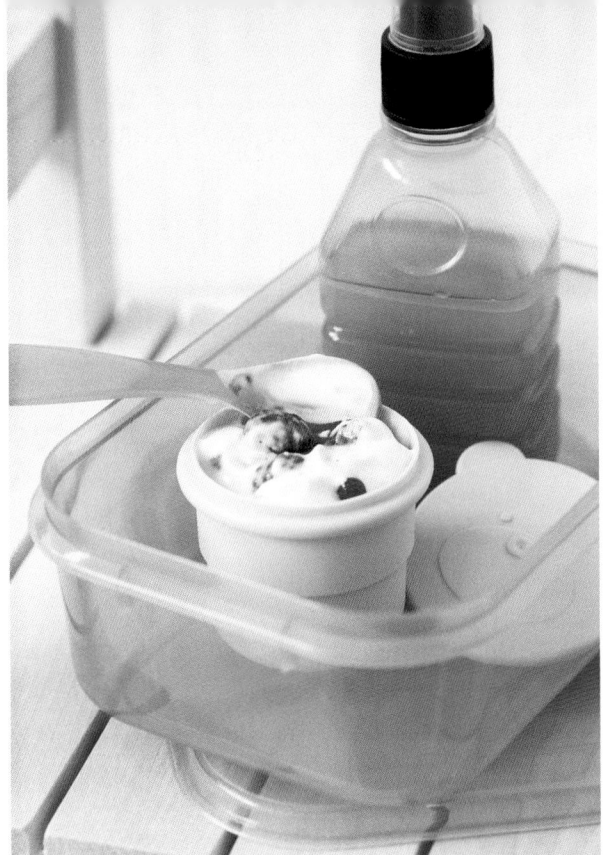

mixed berry yogurt

MAKES APPROXIMATELY 1 CUP

Combine ⅓ cup frozen mixed berries and ¾ cup natural or vanilla yogurt in small bowl.

honey yogurt

MAKES APPROXIMATELY 1 CUP

Combine 1 teaspoon honey and 1 cup natural or vanilla yogurt in small bowl.

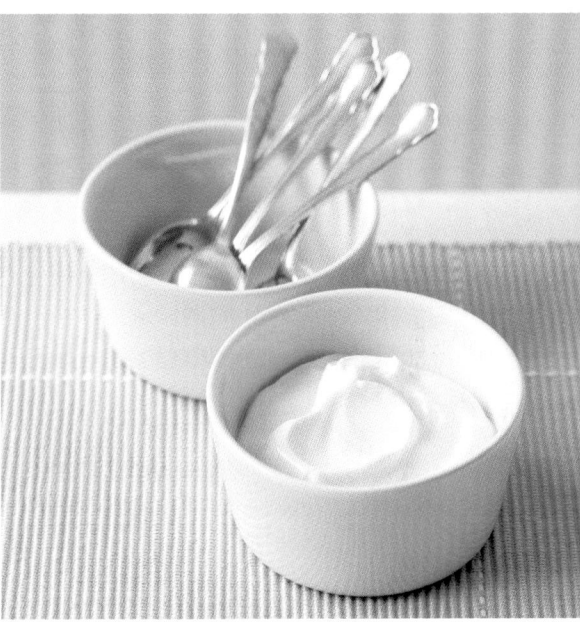

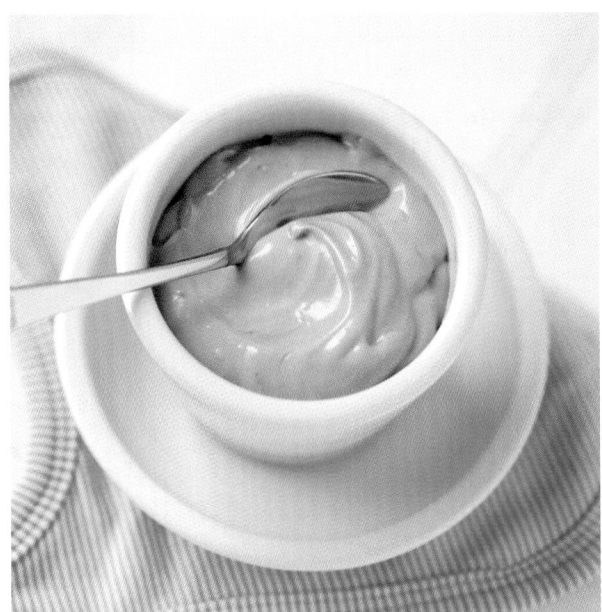

chocolate yogurt

MAKES APPROXIMATELY 1 CUP

Gradually stir 1 cup vanilla yogurt into 50g melted milk eating chocolate in small bowl.

TIP Be careful when adding the yogurt to the chocolate as the mixture can seize if it is added too quickly.

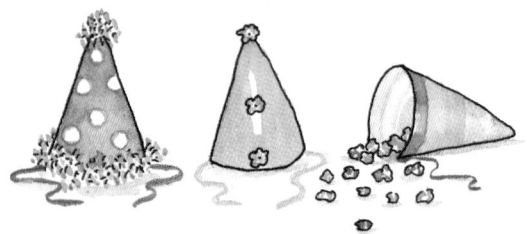

PARTY FOOD

Finger food is ideal for parties, especially when your guests are a band of marauding toddlers who want to eat on the run! As well as being delicious, these recipes will delight the kids.

mini beef rissoles

PREPARATION TIME **25 MINUTES** COOKING TIME **20 MINUTES** MAKES **30**

1kg lean beef mince

1 cup (70g) stale breadcrumbs

½ cup (40g) coarsely grated parmesan

2 cloves garlic, crushed

2 green onions, sliced thinly

1 tablespoon worcestershire sauce

2 tablespoons barbecue sauce

1 tablespoon olive oil

1 Using hand, combine beef, breadcrumbs, cheese, garlic, onion and sauces in large bowl; shape rounded tablespoons of the mixture into rissoles.
2 Heat oil in large non-stick frying pan; cook rissoles, in batches, until cooked through. Drain on absorbent paper.
3 Serve rissoles with tomato sauce, if desired.

TIP You could omit the green onions and replace them with ¼ cup finely chopped fresh flat-leaf parsley, if desired.

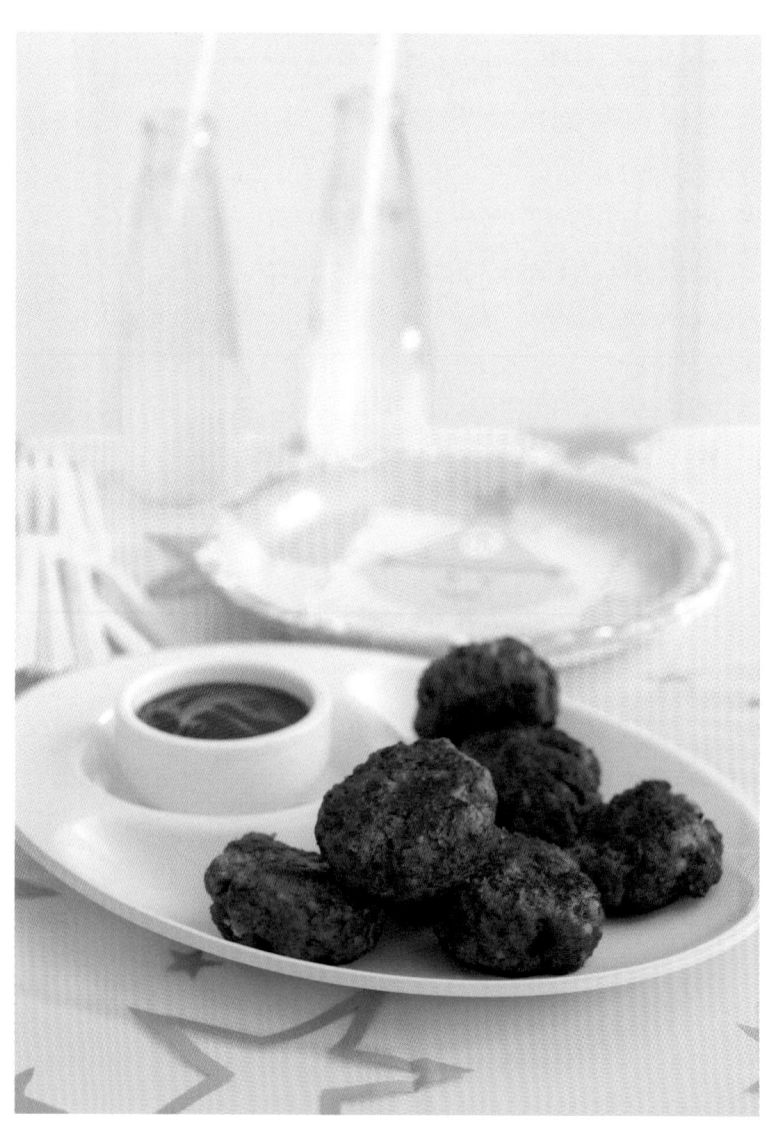

chicken and vegetable rolls

PREPARATION TIME 15 MINUTES   COOKING TIME 30 MINUTES   MAKES 36

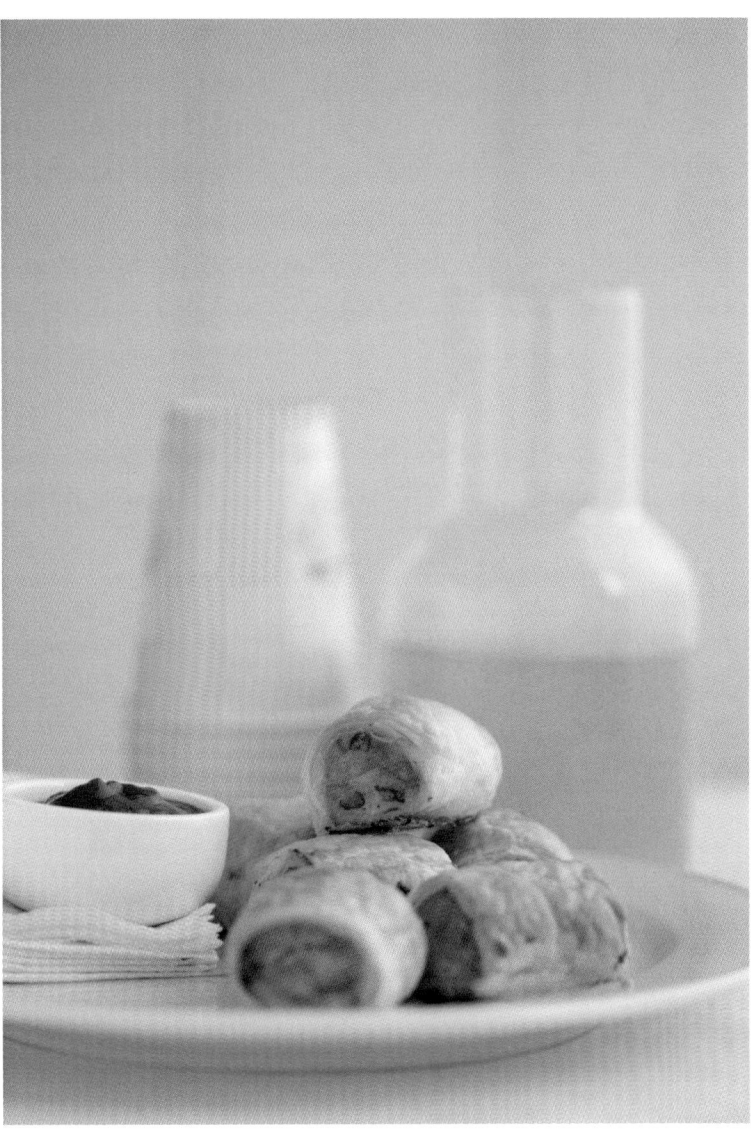

500g chicken mince

1 clove garlic, crushed

1 medium brown onion (150g),
chopped finely

1 medium carrot (120g),
chopped finely

100g green beans, trimmed,
chopped finely

125g can creamed corn

1 egg, beaten lightly

⅓ cup (25g) stale breadcrumbs

1 tablespoon tomato sauce

3 sheets ready-rolled puff pastry

1 egg, beaten lightly, extra

1 Preheat oven to moderately
hot. Oil two oven trays.

2 Using hand, combine mince,
garlic, onion, carrot, beans,
corn, egg, breadcrumbs and
sauce in large bowl.

3 Cut pastry sheets in half
lengthways. Place equal
amounts of chicken mixture
lengthways along centre of
each pastry piece; roll each
pastry piece, from one wide
edge, to enclose filling. Cut
each roll into six pieces.

4 Place, seam-side down, on
prepared trays; brush with
extra egg. Bake, uncovered,
in moderately hot oven about
30 minutes or until browned
lightly and cooked through.

TIP Serve with tomato or
barbecue sauce.

barbecue pizzas

PREPARATION TIME 20 MINUTES
COOKING TIME 10 MINUTES MAKES 15

30cm (300g) frozen ready-made pizza base, thawed
2 tablespoons barbecue sauce
½ cup (80g) finely shredded barbecued chicken
⅓ cup (40g) coarsely grated cheddar

1 Preheat oven to moderately hot.
2 Using 5cm-square cutter, cut shapes from pizza base; place bases on oven trays.
3 Divide sauce among bases; top with chicken and cheese. Cook, uncovered, in moderately hot oven about 10 minutes or until brown and crisp.

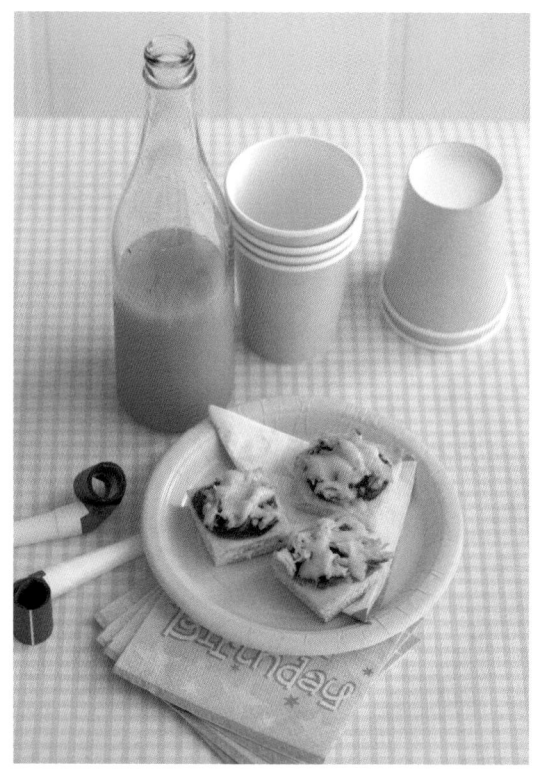

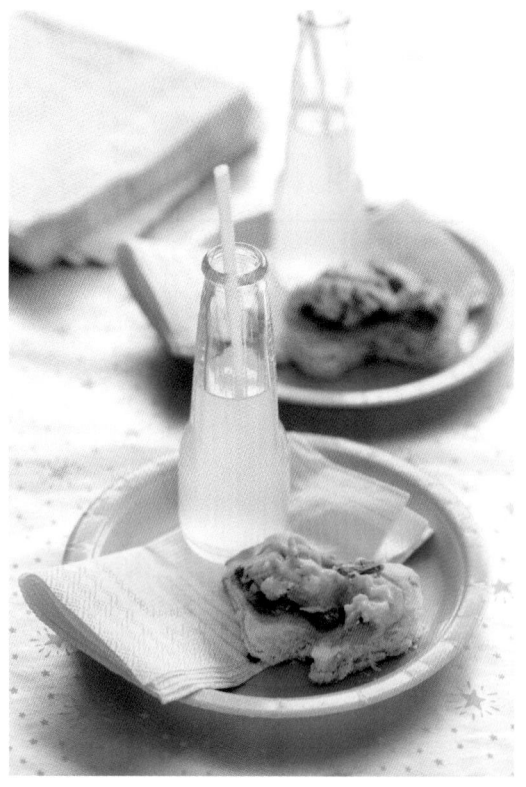

aussie pizzas

PREPARATION TIME 20 MINUTES
COOKING TIME 15 MINUTES MAKES 15

1 bacon rasher (70g), rind removed, sliced thinly
1 egg, beaten lightly
⅓ cup (35g) coarsely grated pizza cheese
30cm (300g) frozen ready-made pizza base, thawed
2 tablespoons bottled tomato pasta sauce

1 Preheat oven to moderately hot.
2 Heat small frying pan; cook bacon, stirring, until crisp. Add egg; cook, stirring, until egg just sets. Remove from heat; stir in cheese.
3 Using 5cm Australia-shape cutter, cut shapes from pizza base; place bases on oven trays.
4 Divide sauce among bases; top with bacon mixture. Cook, uncovered, in moderately hot oven about 10 minutes or until brown and crisp.

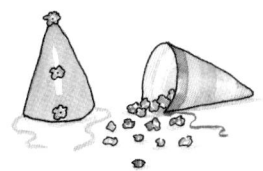

vegetarian pizzas

PREPARATION TIME **20 MINUTES**
COOKING TIME **10 MINUTES** MAKES **15**

30cm (300g) frozen ready-made pizza base, thawed
2 tablespoons tomato paste
⅓ cup (40g) seeded green olives, chopped finely
2 tablespoons finely chopped green capsicum
2 tablespoons finely chopped red capsicum
120g baby bocconcini, chopped finely

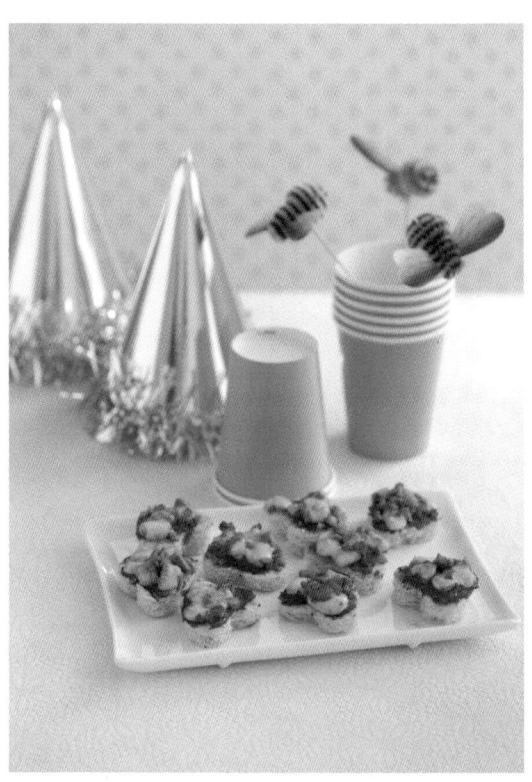

1 Preheat oven to moderately hot.
2 Using 5cm heart-shape cutter, cut shapes from pizza base; place bases on oven trays.
3 Divide paste among bases. Combine olives, capsicums and cheese in small bowl; top pizzas with olive mixture. Cook, uncovered, in moderately hot oven about 10 minutes or until brown and crisp.

salami, mushroom and cheese pizzas

PREPARATION TIME **20 MINUTES**
COOKING TIME **10 MINUTES** MAKES **15**

30cm (300g) frozen ready-made pizza base, thawed
2 tablespoons bottled tomato pasta sauce
10 slices salami (150g), sliced thinly
5 button mushrooms (60g), sliced thickly
5 slices swiss cheese (100g), sliced thinly

1 Preheat oven to moderately hot.
2 Using 5cm-round cutter, cut shapes from pizza base; place bases on oven trays.
3 Divide sauce among bases; top with salami, mushrooms and cheese. Cook, uncovered, in moderately hot oven about 10 minutes or until brown and crisp.

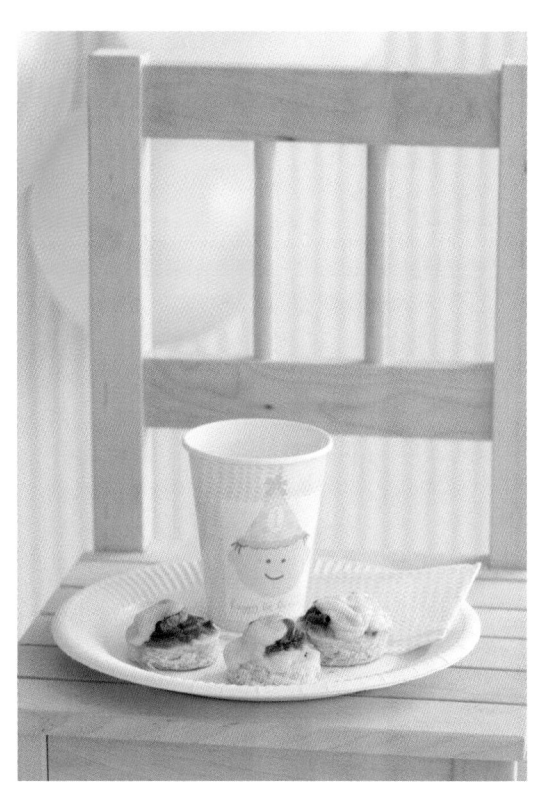

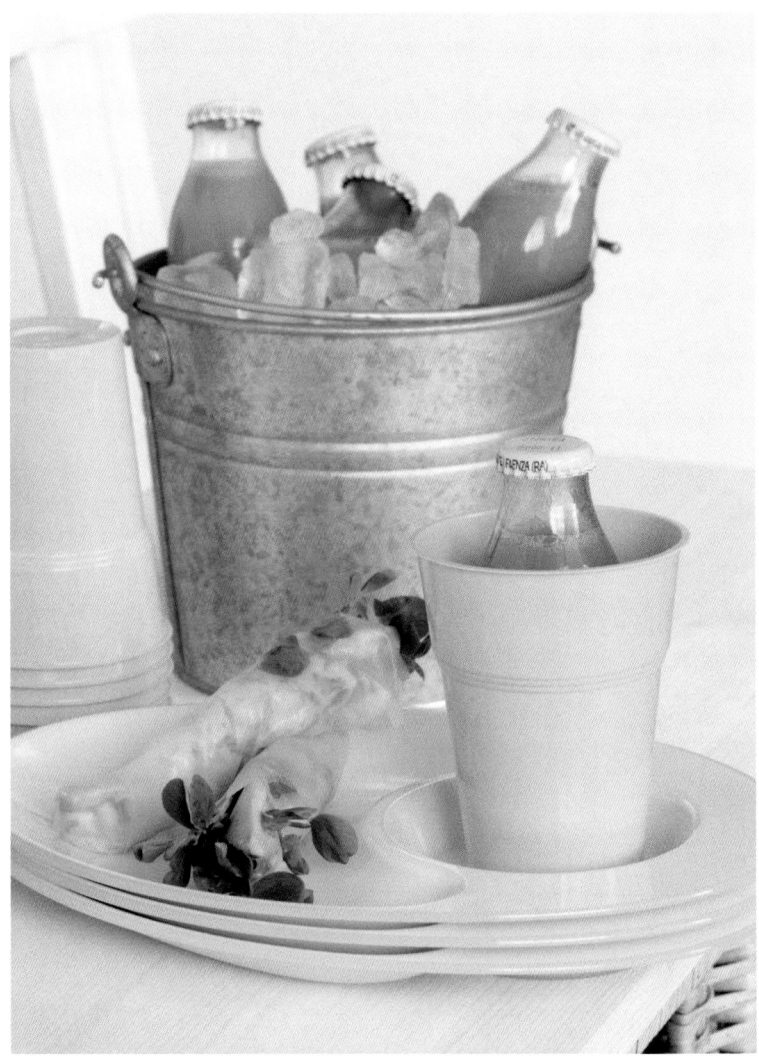

prawn and avocado rice paper rolls

PREPARATION TIME **30 MINUTES**
MAKES **24**

24 cooked medium king
  prawns (1.1kg)

2 tablespoons mayonnaise

24 x 17cm-square rice
  paper sheets

1 large avocado (320g),
  sliced thinly

80g snow pea sprouts, trimmed

1 Shell and devein prawns;
chop coarsely. Combine
prawns and mayonnaise in
small bowl.

2 Place 1 sheet of rice paper
in medium bowl of warm
water until just softened;
lift sheet carefully from water,
placing it on a tea-towel-
covered board with a corner
pointing towards you. Place
1 level tablespoon of the
prawn mixture horizontally in
centre of rice paper; top with
a little of the avocado then
a few sprouts. Fold corner
facing you over filling; roll
rice paper to enclose filling,
folding in one side after
first complete turn of roll.
Repeat with remaining rice
paper sheets, prawn mixture,
avocado and sprouts.

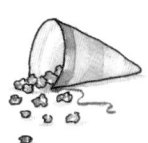

teriyaki chicken rice paper rolls

PREPARATION TIME **30 MINUTES (PLUS REFRIGERATION TIME)**
COOKING TIME **10 MINUTES** MAKES **24**

6 chicken thigh fillets (660g), trimmed

¼ cup (60ml) thick teriyaki marinade

2 tablespoons water

2 lebanese cucumbers (260g)

2 teaspoons peanut oil

24 x 17cm-square rice paper sheets

200g enoki mushrooms, trimmed

1 Slice each chicken thigh into eight strips lengthways. Combine chicken, teriyaki and the water in small bowl, cover; refrigerate 1 hour. Drain chicken; discard marinade.

2 Meanwhile, cut cucumbers in half lengthways; discard seeds. Cut cucumber halves in half crossways; cut pieces into three strips lengthways.

3 Heat oil in large frying pan; cook chicken, in batches, until cooked through. Cool 10 minutes.

4 Place 1 sheet of rice paper in medium bowl of warm water until just softened; lift sheet carefully from water, placing it on a tea-towel-covered board with a corner pointing towards you. Place two pieces of chicken horizontally in centre of rice paper; top with one piece of cucumber then a few mushrooms. Fold corner facing you over filling; roll rice paper to enclose filling, folding in one side after first complete turn of roll. Repeat with remaining rice paper sheets, chicken, cucumber and mushrooms.

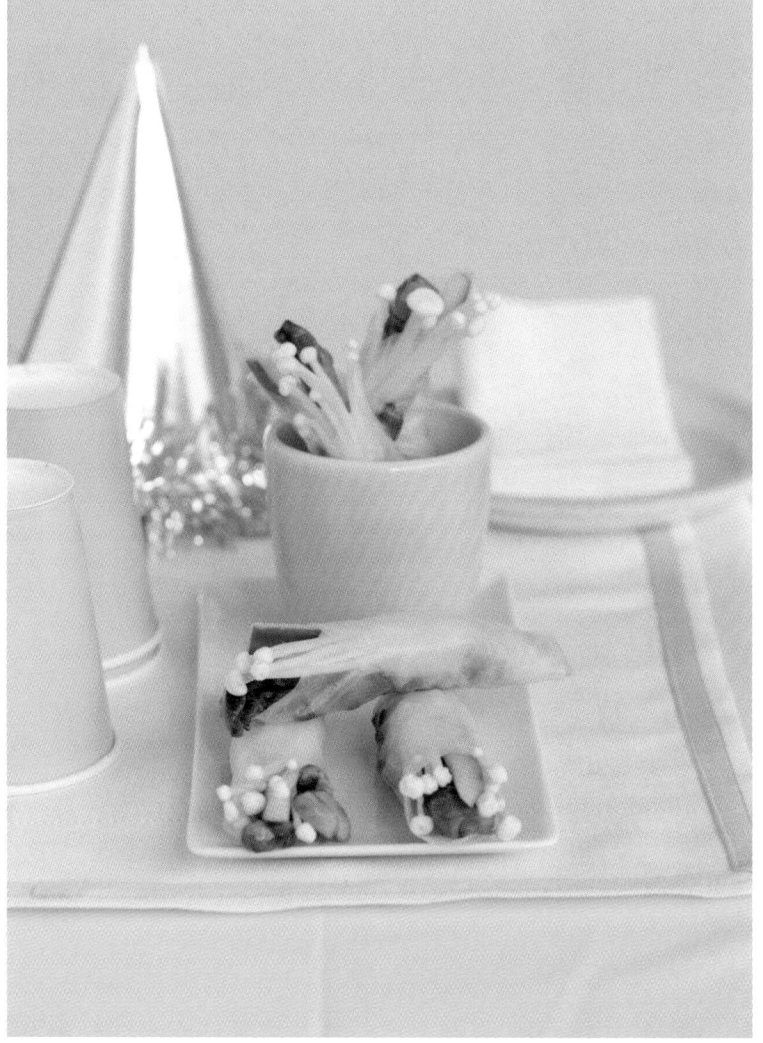

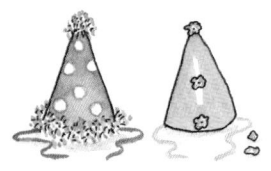

vegetable rice paper rolls

PREPARATION TIME **30 MINUTES** COOKING TIME **5 MINUTES** MAKES **24**

1 large carrot (180g);
   grated coarsely

2 trimmed celery sticks (200g),
   chopped finely

150g chinese cabbage,
   shredded finely

2 teaspoons fish sauce

2 teaspoons brown sugar

1 tablespoon lemon juice

24 x 17cm-square rice
   paper sheets

24 fresh mint leaves

1 Combine carrot, celery, cabbage, sauce, sugar and juice in small bowl.

2 Place 1 sheet of rice paper in medium bowl of warm water until just softened; lift sheet carefully from water, placing it on a tea-towel-covered board with a corner pointing towards you. Place 1 level tablespoon of the vegetable mixture horizontally in centre of sheet; top with 1 mint leaf. Fold corner facing you over filling; roll rice paper to enclose filling, folding in sides after first complete turn of roll. Repeat with remaining rice paper sheets, vegetable mixture and mint leaves.

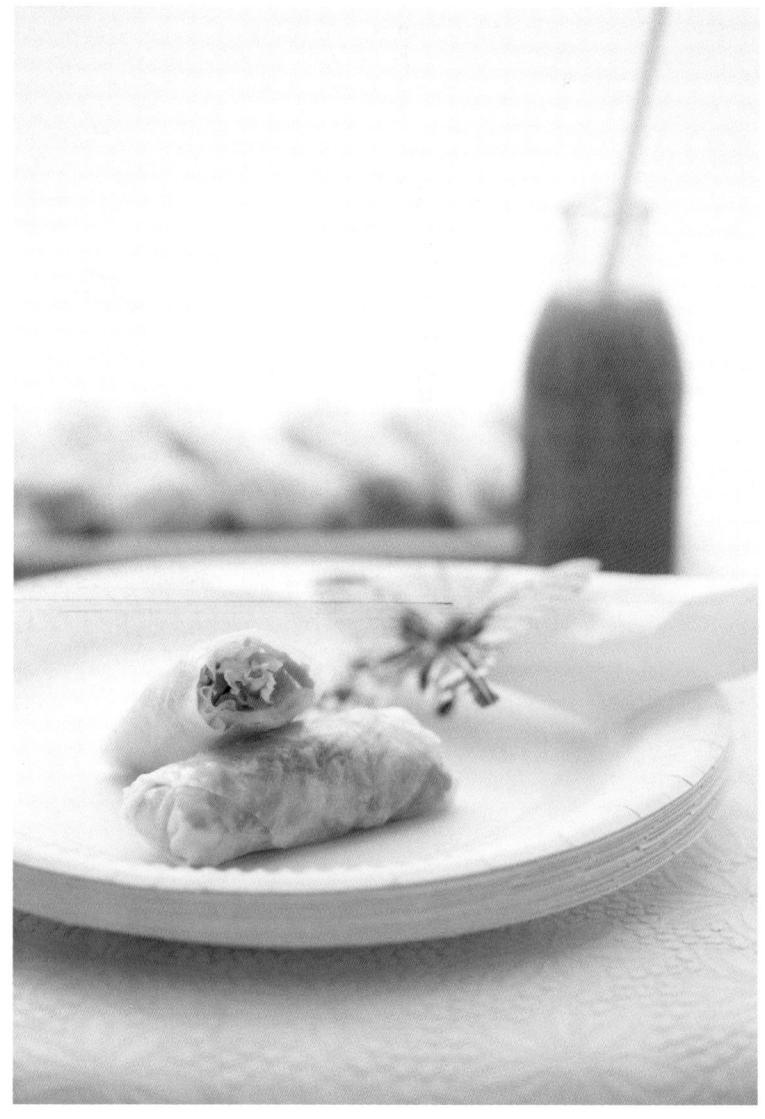

tofu and bok choy rice paper rolls

PREPARATION TIME 30 MINUTES   COOKING TIME 5 MINUTES   MAKES 24

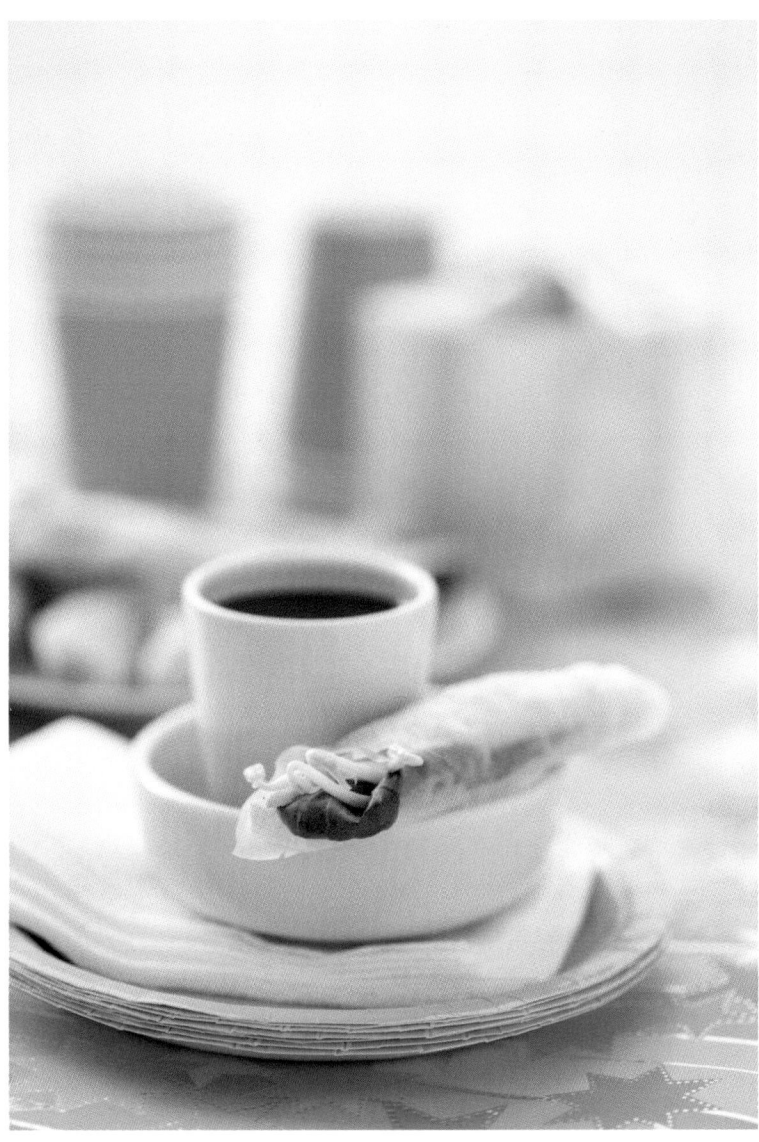

12 fresh baby corn,
    halved horizontally

24 baby bok choy leaves

300g firm silken tofu

2 cups (160g) bean sprouts

24 x 17cm-square rice
    paper sheets

CHILLI SAUCE

⅓ cup (80ml) sweet chilli sauce

1 tablespoon soy sauce

1 Boil, steam or microwave corn and bok choy, separately, until tender; drain.

2 Meanwhile, combine ingredients for chilli sauce in small bowl.

3 Halve tofu horizontally; cut each half into 12 even strips. Place tofu in medium bowl with half of the chilli sauce.

4 Place 1 sheet of rice paper in medium bowl of warm water until just softened; lift sheet carefully from water, placing it on a tea-towel-covered board with a corner pointing towards you. Place one tofu strip horizontally in centre of sheet; top with one piece of corn then a bok choy leaf and a few sprouts. Fold corner facing you over filling; roll rice paper to enclose filling, folding in one side after first complete turn of roll. Repeat with remaining rice paper sheets, tofu, corn, bok choy and sprouts. Serve rolls with remaining chilli sauce.

chicken and creamed corn sandwiches

PREPARATION TIME **10 MINUTES** MAKES **12**

1¼ cups (200g) finely chopped cooked chicken

125g can creamed corn

8 slices wholemeal bread

2 tablespoons mayonnaise

1 cup (60g) coarsely shredded iceberg lettuce

1 Combine chicken and corn in medium bowl.
2 Spread four slices of the bread with mayonnaise; top with chicken mixture and lettuce then remaining bread slices. Discard crusts; cut sandwiches into fingers.

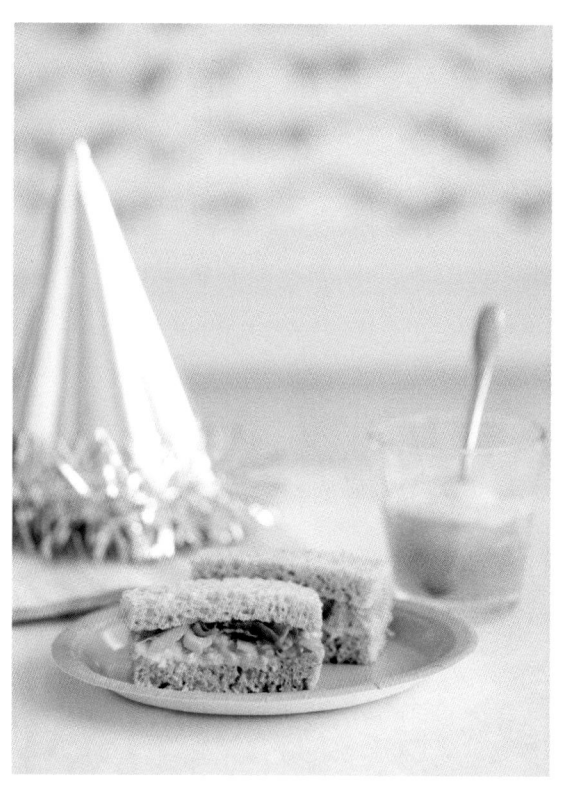

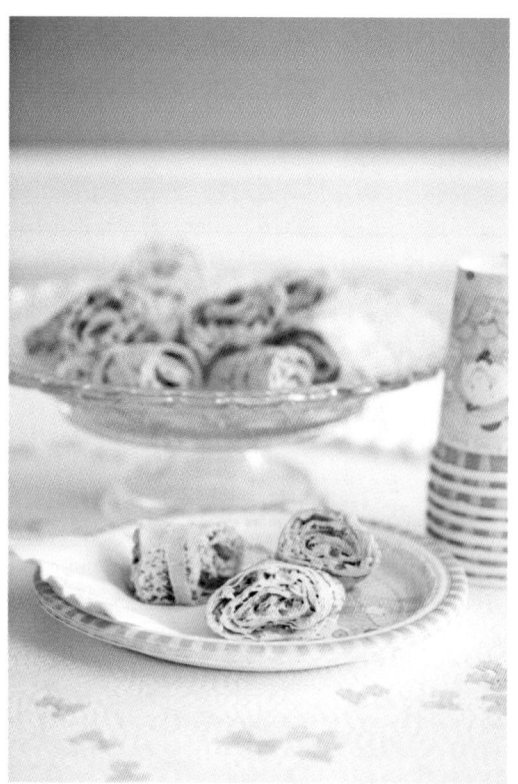

tuna and carrot pinwheels

PREPARATION TIME **20 MINUTES** MAKES **12**

185g can tuna in brine, drained

1 small carrot (70g), grated finely

2 gherkins (40g), chopped finely

¼ cup (75g) mayonnaise

6 slices lavash

2 tablespoons mayonnaise, extra

1 Combine tuna, carrot, gherkins and mayonnaise in medium bowl.
2 Spread one slice of bread with ⅓ of the extra mayonnaise; top with another piece of bread. Spread ⅓ of the tuna mixture along short edge of bread. Roll bread tightly; trim edges. Using serrated knife, cut roll into four pieces. Repeat with remaining bread, extra mayonnaise and tuna mixture.

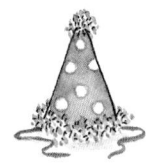

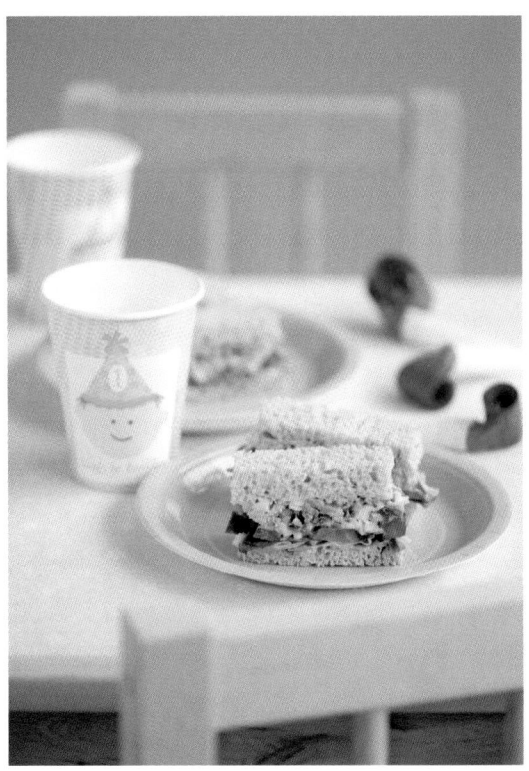

blt

PREPARATION TIME 20 MINUTES   COOKING TIME 5 MINUTES
MAKES 12

2 bacon rashers (140g), rind removed, chopped finely
2 hard-boiled eggs, chopped finely
¼ cup (75g) mayonnaise
½ cup (30g) coarsely shredded butter lettuce
1 small tomato (90g), sliced thinly
8 slices wholemeal bread

1   Cook bacon in small heated frying pan, stirring,
    until browned and crisp; drain on absorbent paper.
2   Combine bacon with egg and 2 tablespoons of the
    mayonnaise in small bowl.
3   Divide remaining mayonnaise, lettuce and tomato
    among four slices of the bread; top with egg
    mixture and remaining bread slices. Discard
    crusts; cut sandwiches into fingers.

ricotta and honey sandwiches

PREPARATION TIME 10 MINUTES   MAKES 12

½ cup (100g) ricotta
1 tablespoon honey
¼ cup (35g) dried pears, chopped finely
6 slices raisin bread

1   Combine ricotta, honey and pear in small bowl.
2   Divide ricotta mixture among three slices of the
    bread; top with remaining bread slices. Discard
    crusts; cut sandwiches into squares.

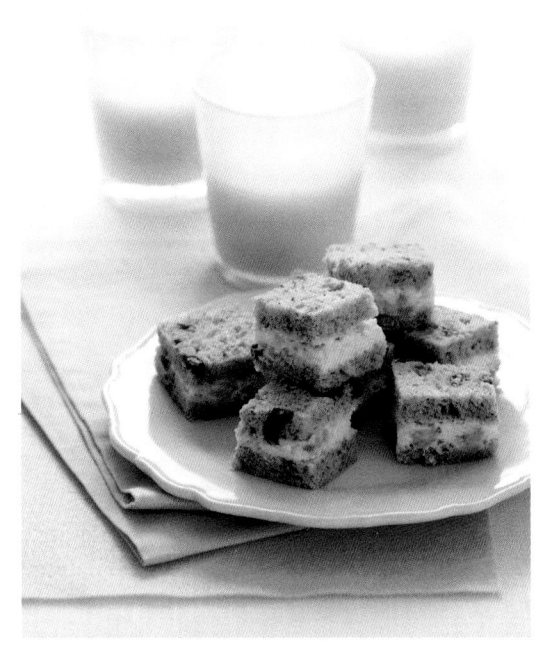

cheesy pastry twists

PREPARATION TIME 20 MINUTES
COOKING TIME 10 MINUTES MAKES 24

2 sheets ready-rolled puff
    pastry, thawed
1 egg yolk, beaten
1 cup (100g) coarsely grated
    pizza cheese
½ cup (40g) finely grated
    parmesan

1   Preheat oven to moderately
    hot. Oil two oven trays; line
    with baking paper.
2   Brush one pastry sheet with
    half of the egg yolk; sprinkle
    with pizza cheese. Top with
    remaining pastry sheet;
    brush with remaining egg
    yolk. Sprinkle with parmesan
    cheese. Cut pastry stack in
    half; place one pastry half
    on top of the other, pressing
    down firmly to seal.
3   Cut pastry widthways into
    24 strips; twist each, pinching
    ends to seal. Place twists
    on prepared trays; bake,
    uncovered, in moderately
    hot oven about 10 minutes
    or until browned lightly.

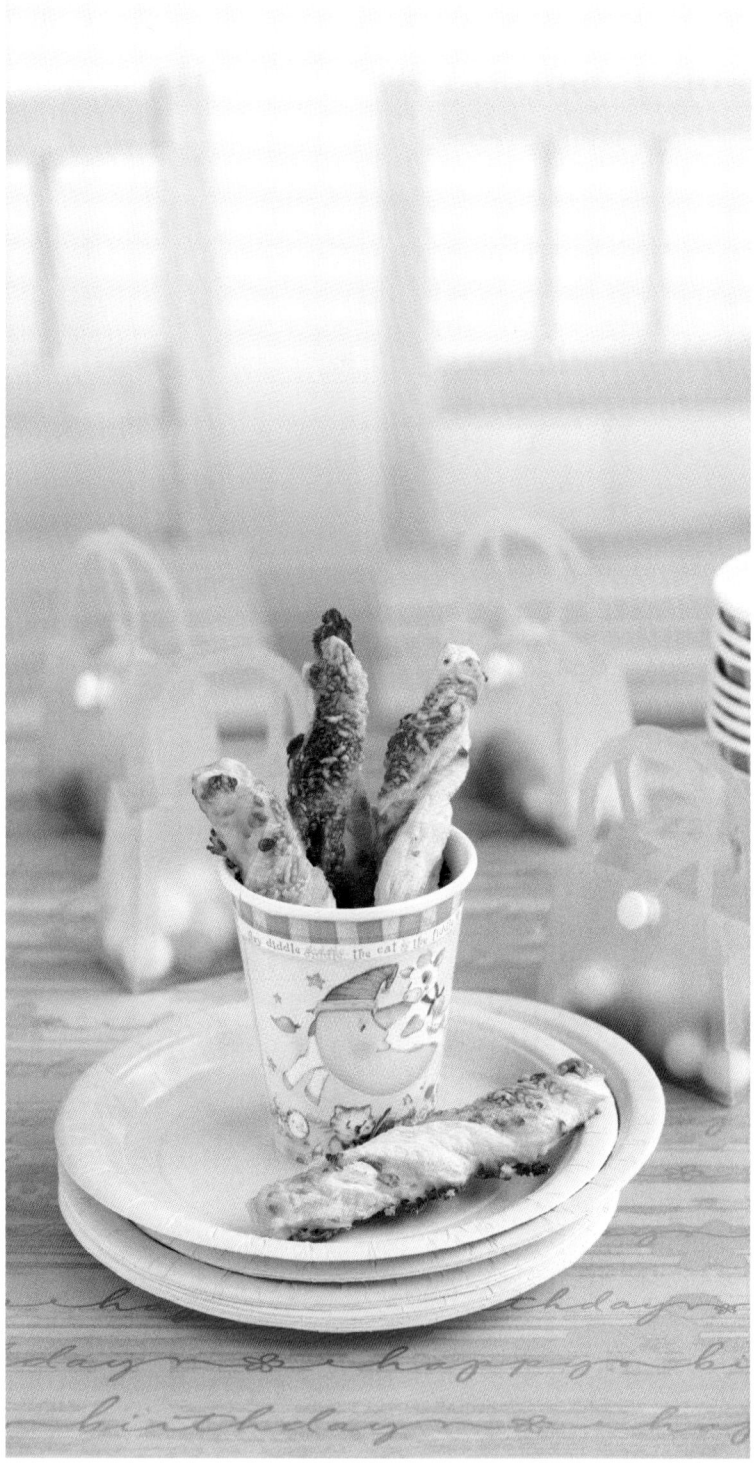

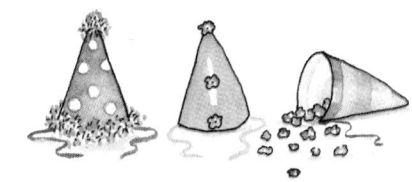

mini chocolate brownie triangles

PREPARATION TIME 15 MINUTES (PLUS STANDING TIME)
COOKING TIME 35 MINUTES MAKES 32

125g butter, chopped

200g dark eating chocolate, chopped coarsely

¾ cup (165g) caster sugar

1 teaspoon vanilla extract

2 eggs, beaten lightly

1 cup (150g) plain flour

1 Preheat oven to moderate. Grease deep 19cm-square cake pan; line base and two sides with baking paper, extending paper 2cm above edges of pan.

2 Stir butter and chocolate in medium heatproof bowl over medium saucepan of simmering water until smooth. Remove from heat; stir in sugar and extract then eggs and flour. Pour mixture into prepared pan; bake, uncovered, in moderate oven about 30 minutes or until just firm. Cool in pan.

3 Turn brownie onto board; cut into 16 squares then halve squares to form triangles.

TIP For an easy sour cream frosting, melt 100g dark eating chocolate and fold it into ¼ cup sour cream.

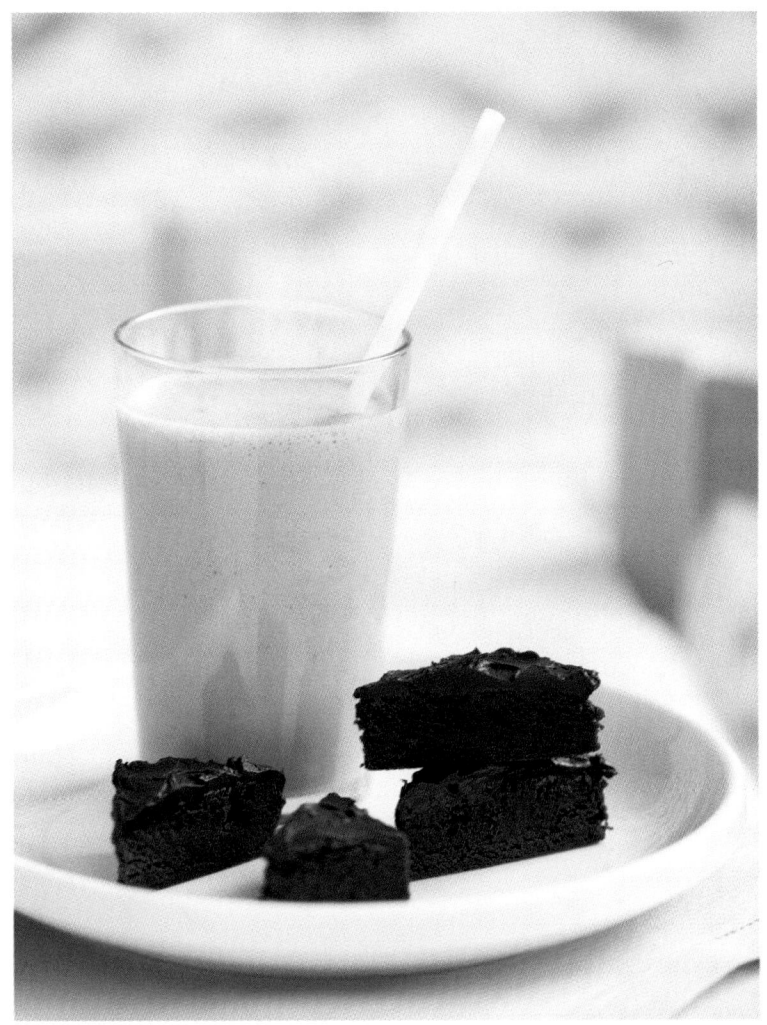

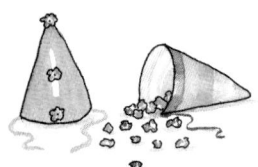

teddy bear biscuits

PREPARATION TIME 35 MINUTES
(PLUS REFRIGERATION TIME)
COOKING TIME 15 MINUTES
MAKES 12

You will need 12 iceblock sticks for this recipe.

200g butter, softened

1 teaspoon vanilla extract

¾ cup (165g) caster sugar

1 egg

40g dark eating chocolate, grated finely

1¼ cups (175g) plain flour

2 tablespoons cocoa powder

24 mini M&M's

12 dark chocolate Melts

1   Preheat oven to moderate. Grease three oven trays; line with baking paper.

2   Beat butter, extract, sugar and egg in small bowl with electric mixer until just changed to a pale colour; do not overbeat. Stir in chocolate, sifted flour and cocoa. Refrigerate 15 minutes.

3   Roll 24 level teaspoons of the mixture into balls. Roll remaining mixture into 12 large balls for teddy faces. On each tray, flatten four large balls with palm of hand to form an 8cm diameter circle. Position two small balls on top of each circle for ears.

Flatten balls with palm of hand. Slide one iceblock stick two-thirds of the way into dough on each face.

4   Position M&M's into dough for eyes and Melts for nose. Bake, uncovered, in moderate oven about 12 minutes or until browned lightly. Cool on trays.

TIP Biscuits can be stored in an airtight container.

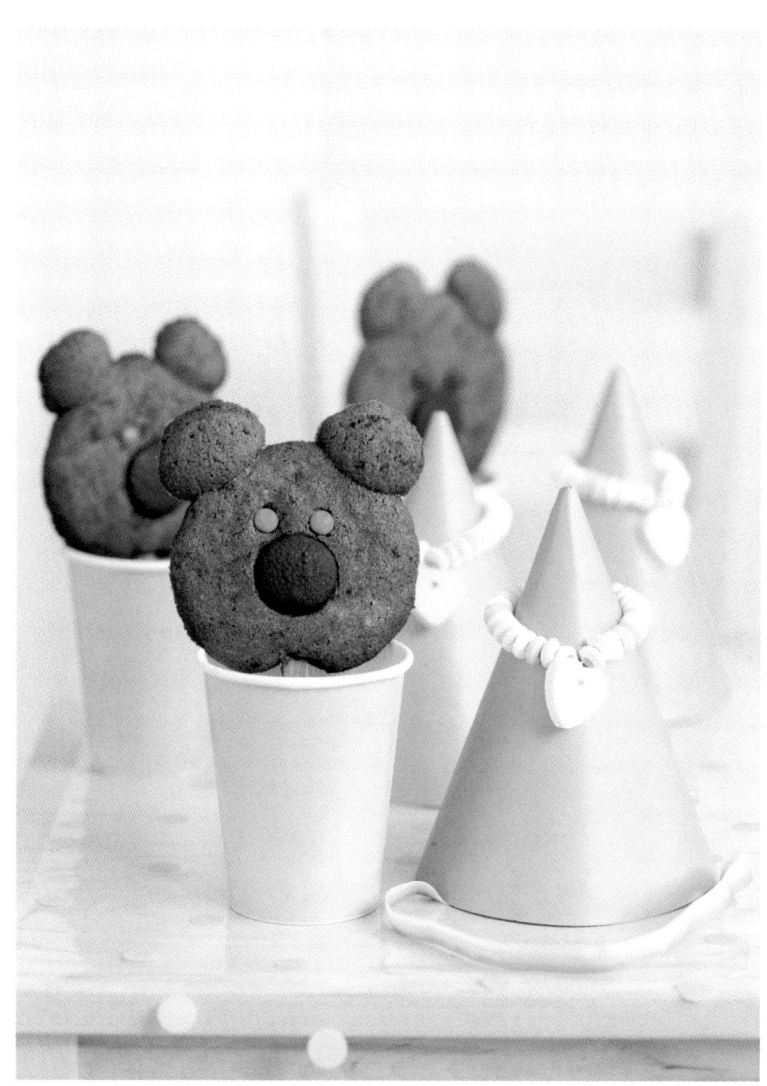

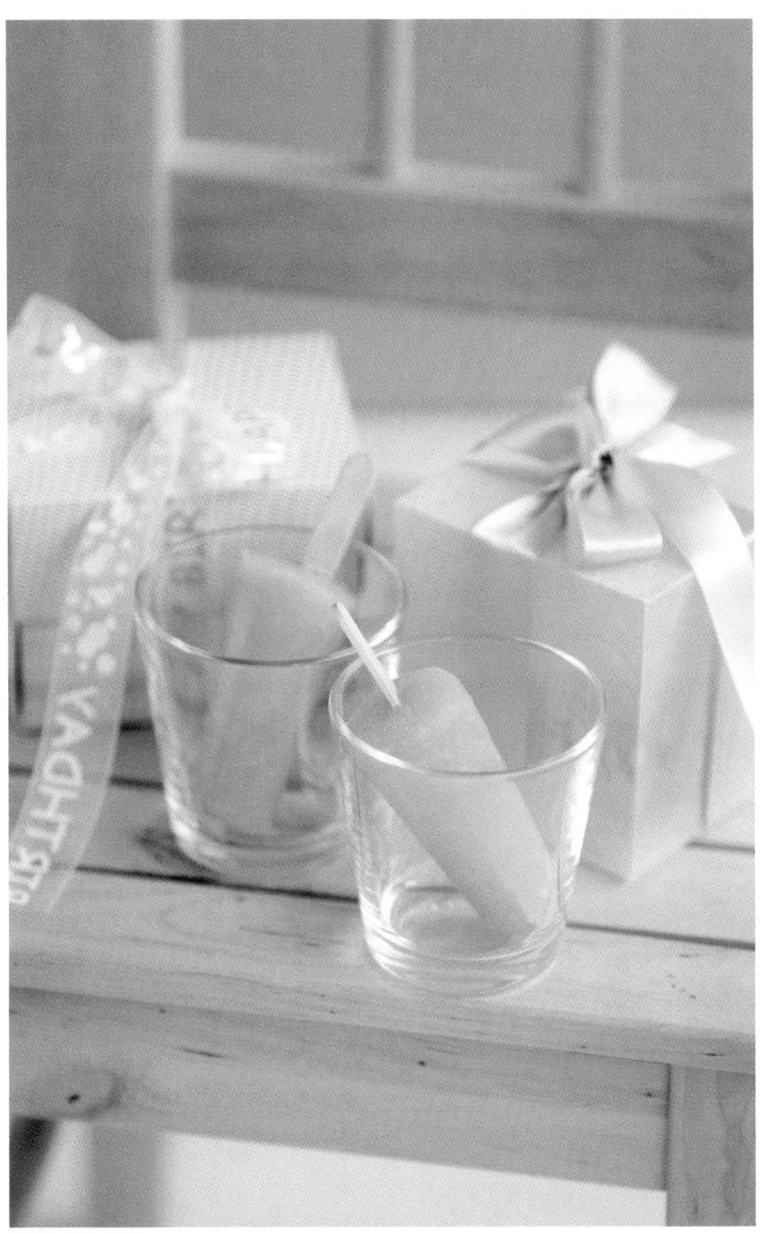

mango, pineapple and orange ice-blocks

PREPARATION TIME **20 MINUTES**
(PLUS FREEZING TIME) MAKES **8**

1 medium pineapple (1.25kg),
  chopped coarsely
1 small mango (300g),
  chopped coarsely
½ cup (125ml) orange juice

1 Blend or process pineapple
   and mango until smooth.
   Using wooden spoon, push
   pineapple mixture through
   fine sieve or mouli into large
   bowl. Stir in juice.
2 Pour pineapple mixture into
   8 x ⅓-cup (80ml) ice-block
   moulds. Freeze 3 hours or
   until firm.

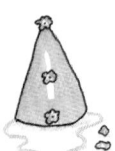

white chocolate crackles

PREPARATION TIME **10 MINUTES (PLUS REFRIGERATION TIME)** MAKES **24**

1 cup (35g) Rice Bubbles
1 cup (35g) Coco Pops
2 x 35g tubes mini M&M's
1 cup (200g) white chocolate
    Melts, melted

1 Line two 12-hole
    (1 tablespoon/20ml)
    mini muffin pans with
    patty-pan cases.
2 Combine ingredients in
    medium bowl. Divide
    mixture among prepared
    holes, cover; refrigerate
    10 minutes.

TIP You need to work quite
quickly when dividing the
mixture among the muffin holes,
as the chocolate sets quickly.

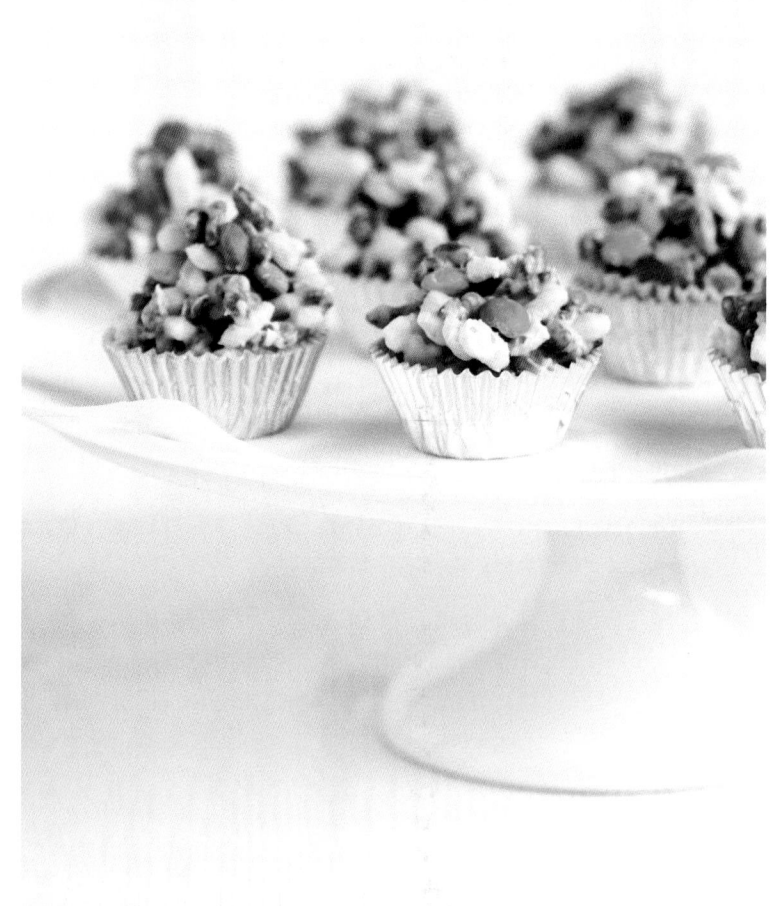

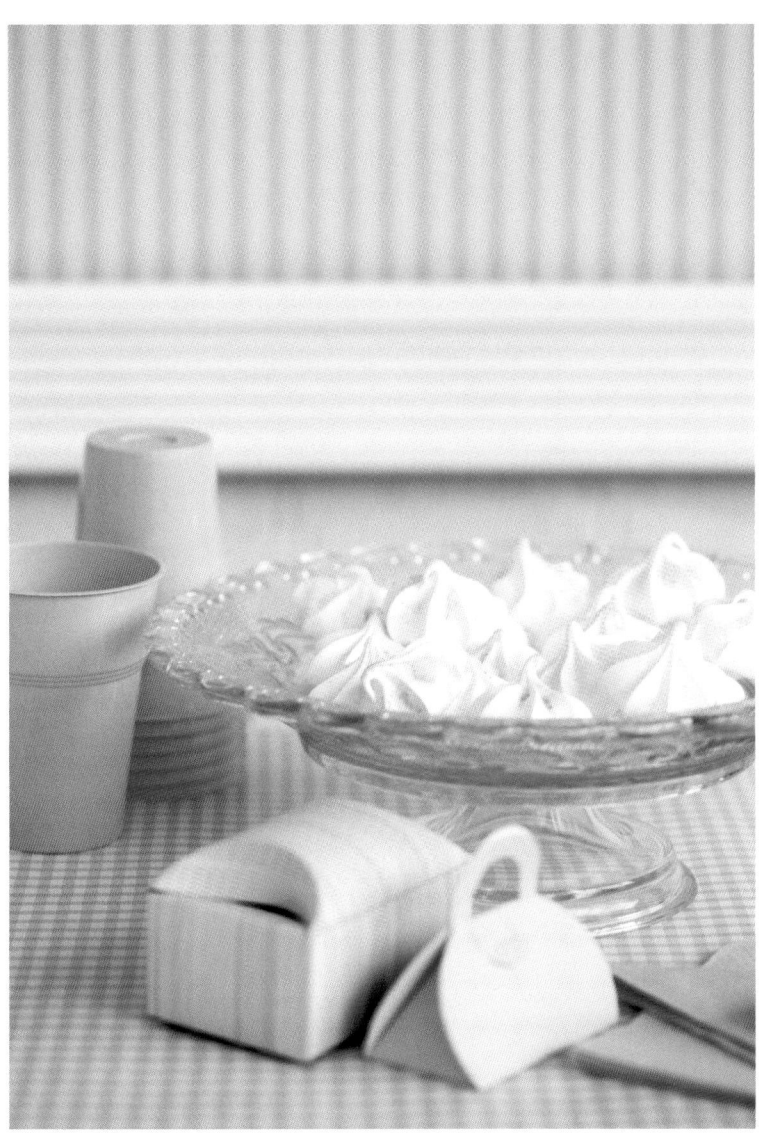

meringue kisses

PREPARATION TIME 15 MINUTES
COOKING TIME 30 MINUTES   MAKES 30

2 teaspoons cornflour
2 egg whites
⅔ cup (150g) caster sugar
1 teaspoon white vinegar
2 teaspoons icing sugar mixture
2 teaspoons caster sugar, extra
assorted food colourings

1 Preheat oven to very slow. Grease two oven trays; dust with cornflour, shake off excess.
2 Beat egg whites in small bowl with electric mixer until soft peaks form. Gradually add caster sugar, 1 tablespoon at a time, beating until sugar dissolves between additions. Fold in vinegar and icing sugar.
3 Place half of the extra caster sugar with a drop of colouring in small plastic bag; rub colouring into sugar until evenly coloured. Repeat with remaining sugar and another colour.
4 Place meringue mixture in piping bag fitted with a 2.5cm-star nozzle; pipe 4cm stars, 3cm apart, on prepared trays. Sprinkle with coloured sugars. Bake, uncovered, in very slow oven about 30 minutes. Cool meringues on trays.

105

BIRTHDAY CAKES

No pressure, but the candlelit birthday cake is the highlight of a toddler's birthday party. Read on for some shining examples...

funny faces

PREPARATION TIME 1 HOUR 20 MINUTES (PLUS COOLING TIME)   COOKING TIME 20 MINUTES

You need a 55g packet of mini M&M's for this recipe.

6 x 5.5cm paper cases

340g packet buttercake mix

125g butter, softened

1½ cups (240g) icing sugar mixture

2 tablespoons milk

ivory, blue, red, green, purple, orange and yellow colouring

black glossy decorating gel

red glossy decorating gel

17 assorted coloured mini M&M's

4 silver or gold cachous

1 Preheat oven to moderate. Line six holes of 12-hole (⅓ cup/80ml) muffin pan with cases.

2 Make cake according to directions on packet; pour ¼ cup mixture into each case. Bake, uncovered, in moderate oven about 20 minutes. Stand cakes in pan 5 minutes; turn onto wire rack to cool.

3 Beat butter in small bowl with electric mixer until as pale as possible. Gradually beat in half of the sugar, milk, then remaining sugar.

4 Tint two-thirds of butter cream with ivory colouring; spread over tops of cakes.

5 Divide remaining butter cream among six bowls; tint each bowl with one of the remaining colourings. Using small spatula, place hair on cakes with coloured butter creams.

6 Position two M&M's on each cake for eyes. Using black and red decorating gel, pipe pupils, eyebrows, noses, freckles, mouths, eyelashes and ears onto cakes as desired.

7 Use cachous and remaining M&M's to decorate faces as desired.

TIP The cake mix is enough to make 12 cakes, so decorate the other six cakes into other funny faces.

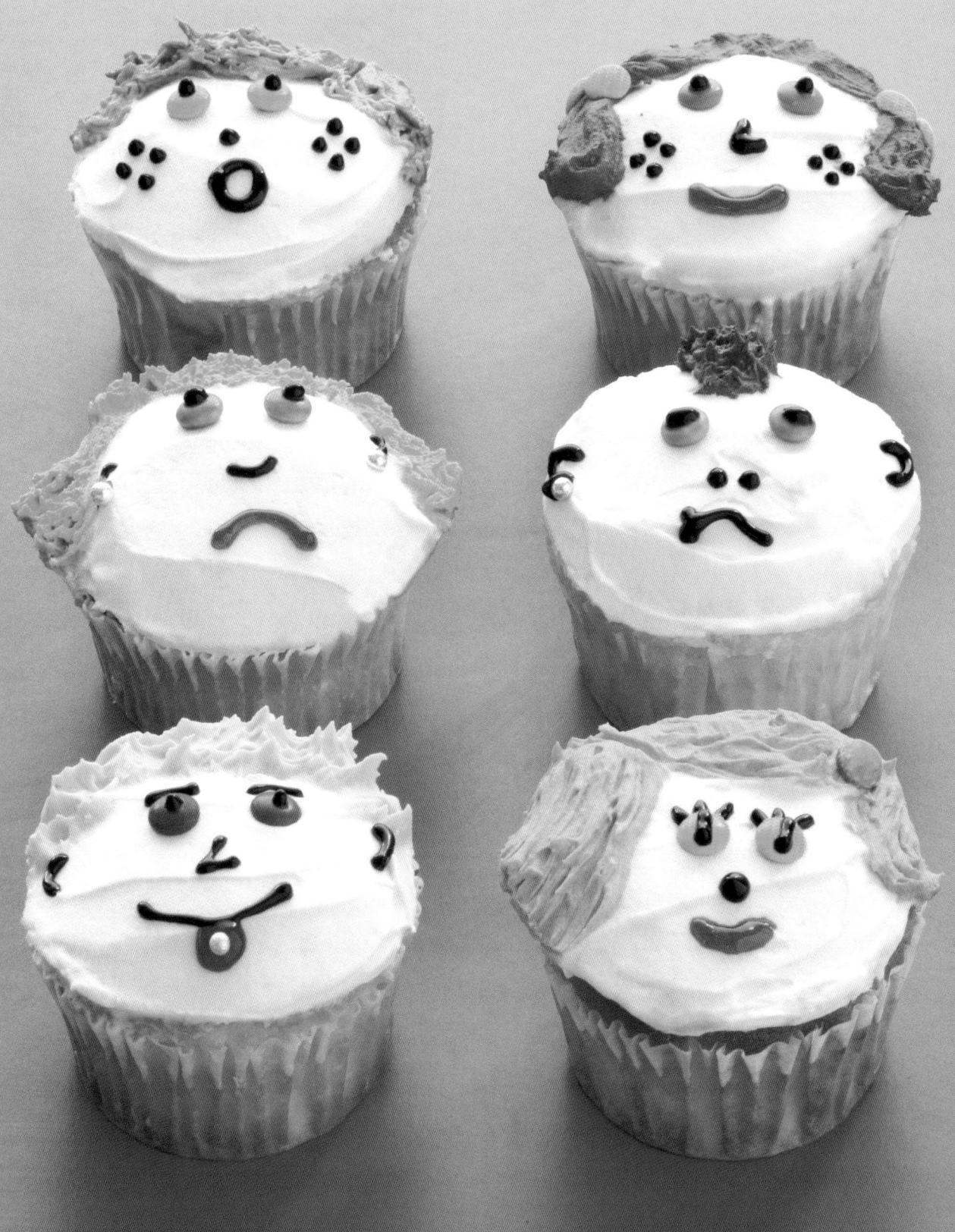

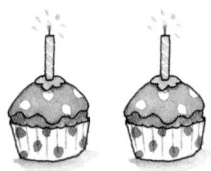

animals

PREPARATION TIME 1 HOUR 20 MINUTES (PLUS COOLING TIME) COOKING TIME 20 MINUTES

6 x 5.5cm paper cases

340g packet buttercake mix

125g butter, softened

1½ cups (240g) icing
   sugar mixture

2 tablespoons milk

black, red, yellow, pink, green
   and orange colouring

1 Preheat oven to moderate. Line six holes of 12-hole (⅓ cup/80ml)
   muffin pan with cases.
2 Make cake according to directions on packet; pour ¼ cup mixture
   into each case. Bake, uncovered, in moderate oven about 20 minutes.
   Stand cakes in pan 5 minutes; turn onto wire rack to cool.
3 Beat butter in small bowl with electric mixer until as pale as possible.
   Gradually beat in half of the sugar, milk, then remaining sugar.
4 Divide butter cream into six portions; tint one portion with just
   enough black to make grey for elephant; tint remaining five portions
   with remaining colours to the strength you prefer.

TIP The cake mix is enough to make 12 cakes so you can decorate
the remaining 6 cakes into other animals of your own choosing.

elephant

1 white marshmallow, halved

2 brown mini M&M's

6cm piece black fresh
   rope licorice

1 white jelly bean, halved

black glossy decorating gel

Spread grey butter cream
over top of one cake. Position
marshmallow halves on cake
for ears. Using any remaining
butter cream, colour insides of
ears. Position M&M's on cake for
eyes, licorice for trunk and jelly
bean halves for tusks. Using gel,
dot pupils onto eyes.

ladybird

1 white marshmallow, halved

2 blue mini M&M's

8cm piece black licorice strap

8 green mini M&M's

black glossy decorating gel

Spread red butter cream
over top of one cake. Position
marshmallow half on cake for
head. Position blue M&M's on
marshmallow for eyes. Cut
licorice strap into thin strips;
position one strip down centre
of cake. Position green M&M's
on cake. Using gel, dot pupils
onto eyes.

fish

7cm piece black licorice strap

2 orange jelly beans

2 fruit salad jellies

1 blue mini M&M

Spread yellow butter cream
over top of one cake. Cut licorice
strap into thin strips; position one
strip on cake as shown. Position
jelly beans on cake for lips. Split
jellies in half horizontally. Position
two halves on cake for tail. Cut
one of the remaining halves
crossways; position on cake
for fin. Using small spatula,
dab butter cream to create fish
scales. Position M&M for eye.

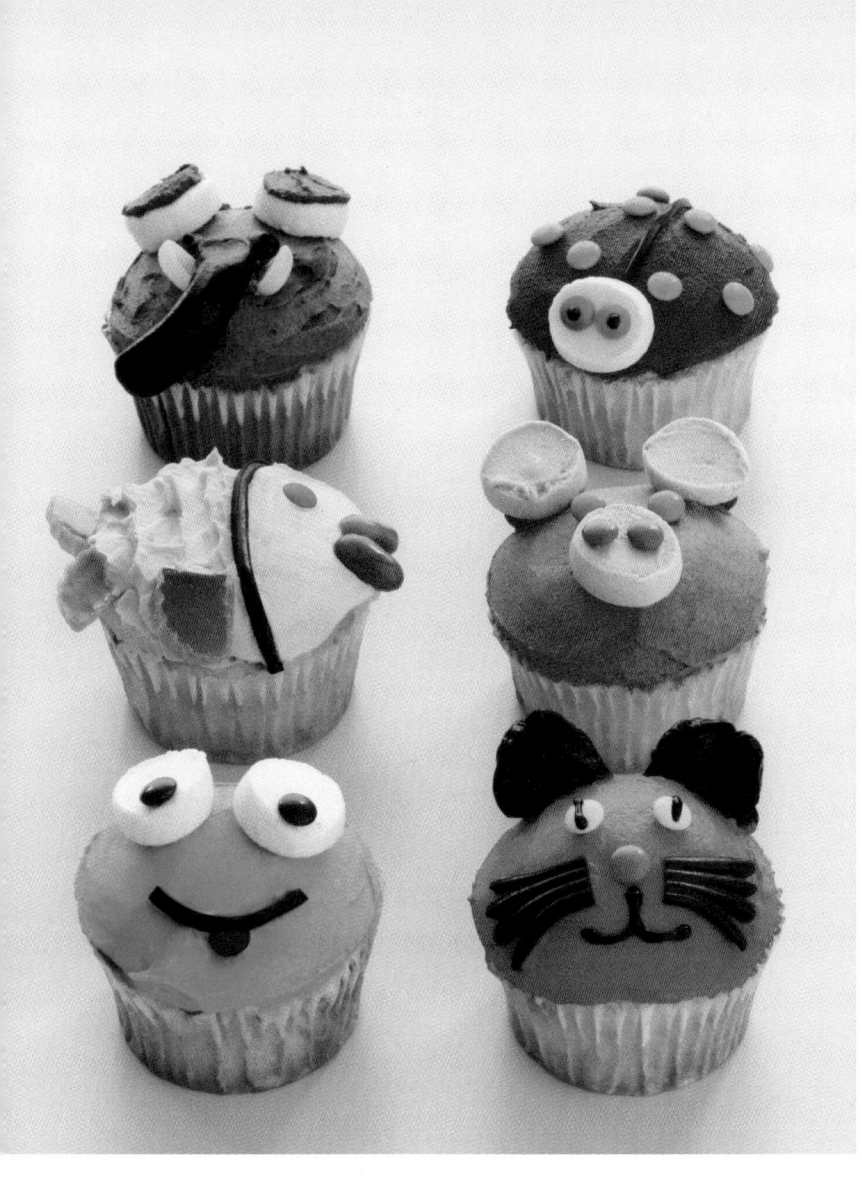

pig

2 pink marshmallows, halved

2 pink mini M&M's

2 blue mini M&M's

Spread pink butter cream over top of one cake. Position one marshmallow half for snout and two halves for ears. Position pink M&M's on marshmallow for nostrils and blue M&M's on cake for eyes.

frog

1 white marshmallow, halved

2 brown mini M&M's

4cm piece black fresh licorice strap

1 red mini M&M, halved

Spread green butter cream over top of one cake. Position marshmallow halves, cut-side up, on cake for eyes. Position brown M&M's on eyes for pupils. Cut licorice strap into thin strips; position one strip on cake for mouth. Position red M&M on cake for tongue.

cat

1 seeded prune, halved

2 yellow mini M&M's

2 x 2.5cm pieces black licorice strap

1 pink mini M&M

black glossy decorating gel

Spread orange butter cream over top of one cake. Position prune halves on cake for ears; position yellow M&M's on cake for eyes. Using gel, draw pupils onto eyes. Cut licorice strap into whiskers; position on cake. Position pink M&M for nose. Using gel, draw mouth onto cake.

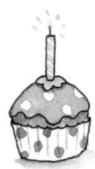

number one

PREPARATION TIME 50 MINUTES (PLUS COOLING TIME) COOKING TIME 30 MINUTES

30 x 2.5cm paper cases

2 x 340g packets buttercake mix

30cm x 40cm cake board

185g butter, softened

2¼ cups (360g) icing
   sugar mixture

¼ cup (60ml) milk

red, purple and orange colouring

6 red licorice straps

4 round chocolate biscuits

1 Preheat oven to moderate. Grease and line 19cm x 29cm slice pan; line 30 holes of three (1 tablespoon/20ml) mini muffin pans with paper cases.

2 Make cake according to directions on packet. Place 1 tablespoon of the mixture in each case; pour remaining mixture into prepared slice pan. Bake mini muffins, uncovered, in moderate oven about 15 minutes and large cake, uncovered, in moderate oven about 30 minutes. Stand cakes 5 minutes; turn onto wire racks to cool.

3 Place large cake on board, top-side down.

4 Beat butter in small bowl with electric mixer until as pale as possible. Gradually beat in half of the sugar, then the milk and finally the remaining sugar.

5 Tint ¾ of the butter cream red. Halve remaining butter cream; tint one half purple and other half orange.

6 Reserve 1 tablespoon of each of the three colours of butter cream. Spread remaining red butter cream all over large cake; spread tops of muffins with remaining two coloured butter creams.

7 Press licorice straps around sides of large cake to form sides of cart. Cut remaining licorice strap lengthways into three strips; plait to form rope. Using toothpick, attach rope to cart.

8 Using a little of the reserved red butter cream, attach biscuits to cart for wheels.

9 Arrange muffins on cart; using reserved purple and orange butter cream, decorate muffin tops with a number 1, the child's name or a birthday message.

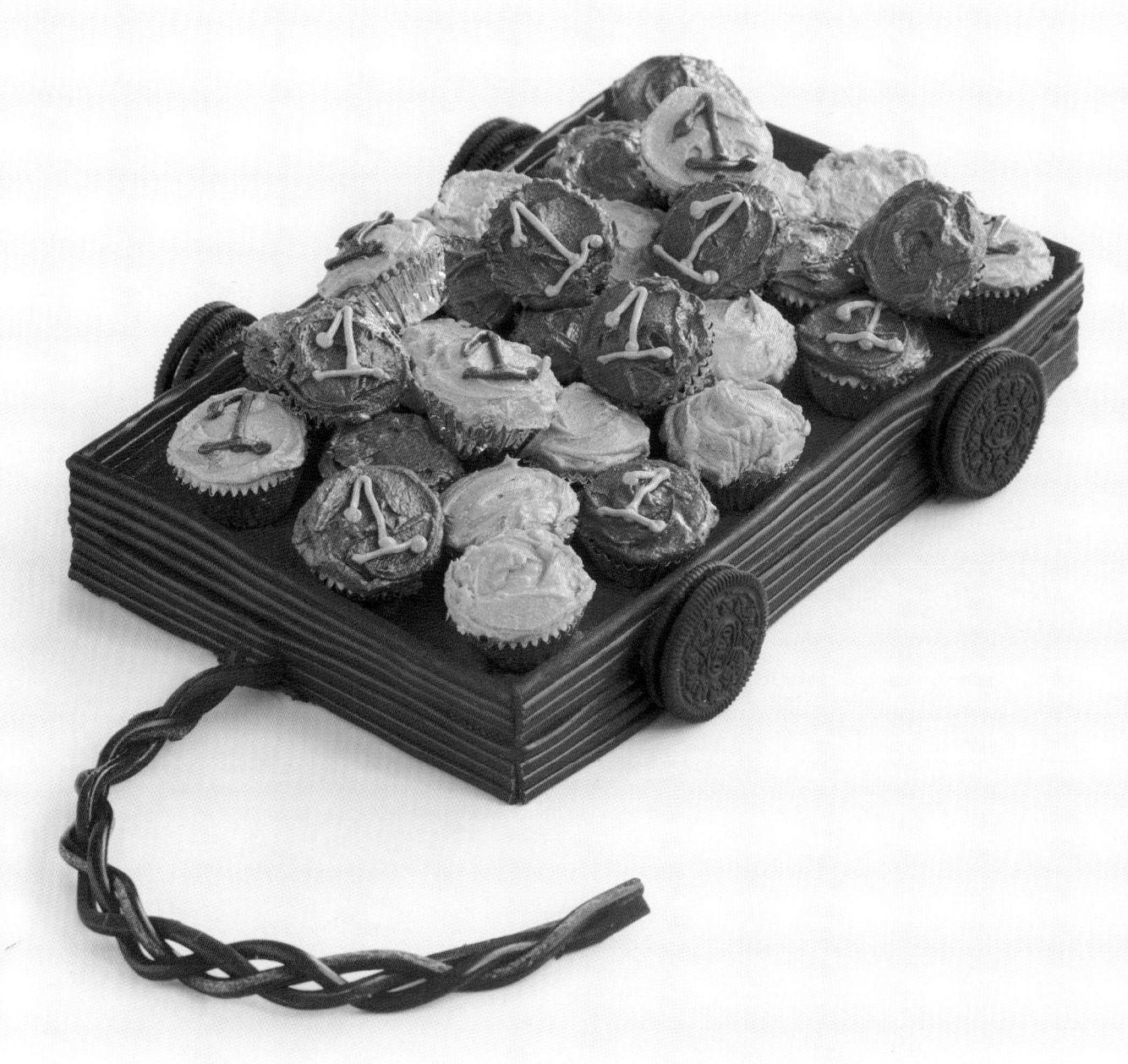

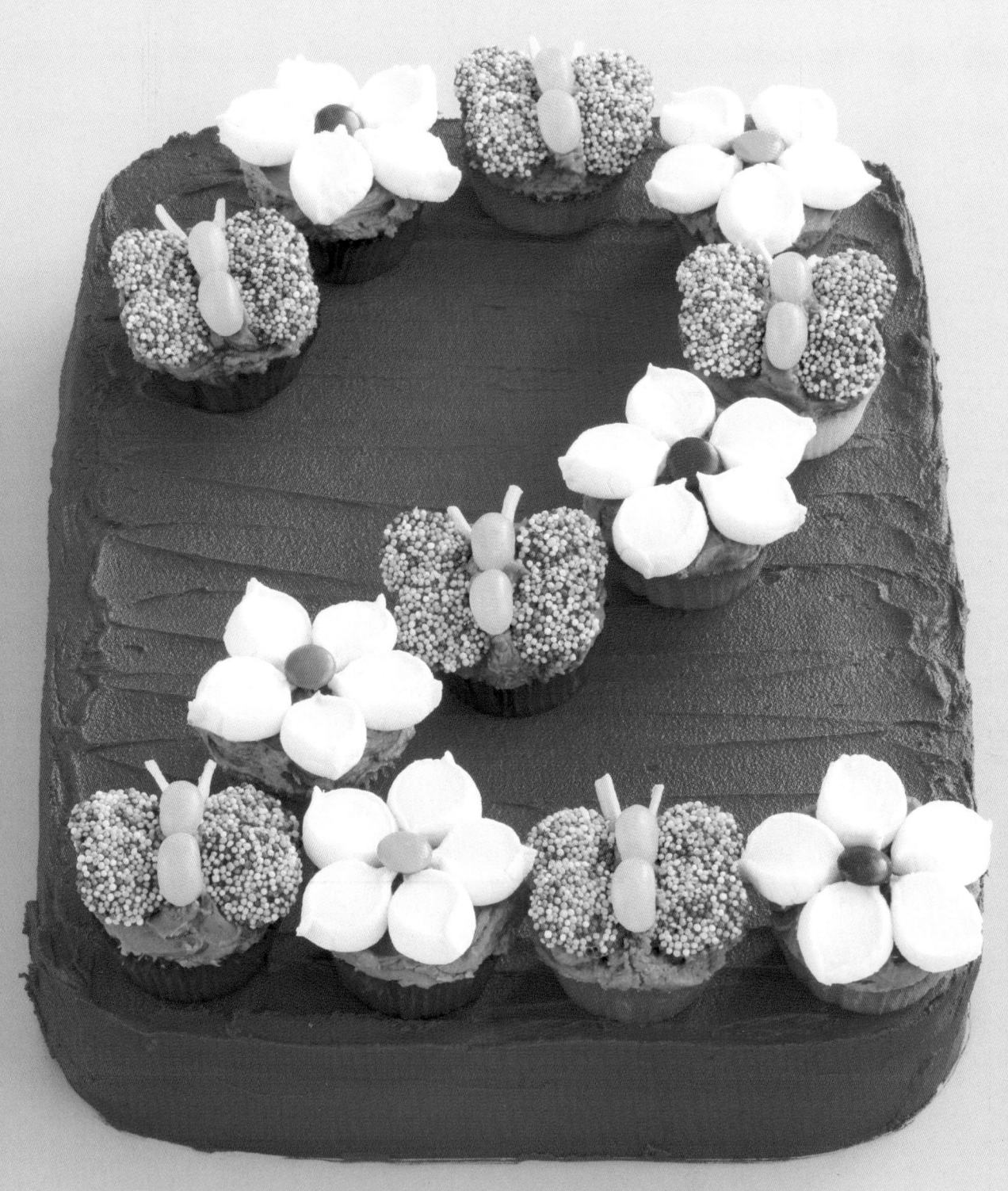

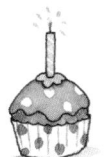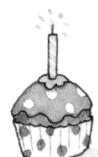

number two

PREPARATION TIME 1 HOUR (PLUS COOLING TIME) COOKING TIME 1 HOUR

12 x 4cm patty-pan cases

3 x 340g packets buttercake mix

35cm x 45cm cake board

250g butter, softened

3 cups (480g) icing sugar mixture

¼ cup (60ml) milk

red and blue colouring

12 yellow jelly beans

24 chocolate freckles

1 yellow Fruit Stick

15 marshmallows

6 Smarties

1 Preheat oven to moderate. Grease and line deep 26cm x 36cm baking dish; line 12-hole (2 tablespoon/40ml) patty pan with cases.

2 Make cake according to directions on packet. Place 2 tablespoons of mixture in each case; pour remaining mixture into prepared dish. Bake patty cakes, uncovered, in moderate oven about 20 minutes and large cake, uncovered, in moderate oven about 1 hour. Stand cakes 5 minutes; turn onto wire racks to cool.

3 Using serrated knife, level top of large cake. Place large cake on board, cut-side down.

4 Beat butter in small bowl with electric mixer until as pale as possible. Gradually beat in half of the sugar, milk, then remaining sugar. Tint two-thirds of the butter cream with red colouring; spread all over large cake. Tint remaining butter cream with blue colouring; spread over tops of patty cakes.

5 Position jelly beans on half of the patty cakes for butterfly bodies; position freckles for butterfly wings. Cut fruit stick into small thin strips; position for butterfly antennae.

6 Using scissors, cut marshmallows in half; squeeze ends of marshmallows together to form petals. Position Smarties on remaining patty cakes for flower buds; position marshmallows for flower petals.

7 Position patty cakes on large cake to form the number 2.

number three

PREPARATION TIME 1 HOUR (PLUS COOLING TIME) COOKING TIME 35 MINUTES

9 x 4cm patty-pan cases

3 x 340g packets buttercake mix

35cm x 45cm cake board

185g butter, softened

2¼ cups (360g) icing
    sugar mixture

2 tablespoons milk

blue and yellow colouring

½ cup (35g) shredded coconut

16 dark pink jelly beans

1 white mallow bake

black glossy decorating gel

5cm piece black licorice strap

1 Preheat oven to moderate. Grease and line two 20cm ring pans;
   line nine holes of 12-hole (2 tablespoon/40ml) patty pan with cases.

2 Make cake according to directions on packet. Place 2 tablespoons
   of mixture in each case; pour remaining mixture into prepared
   ring pans. Bake patty cakes, uncovered, in moderate oven about
   20 minutes and ring cakes, uncovered, in moderate oven about
   35 minutes. Stand cakes 5 minutes; turn onto wire racks to cool.

3 Using serrated knife, level tops of ring cakes. Position ring cakes
   cut-side down; cut segments from cakes, as shown below.
   Assemble cake pieces on board, cut-side down, to form the
   number 3; discard remaining cake.

4 Beat butter in small bowl with electric mixer until as pale as
   possible. Gradually beat in half of the sugar, milk, then remaining
   sugar. Tint ¾ of the butter cream with blue colouring; spread
   all over number cake. Tint remaining butter cream with yellow
   colouring; spread over tops of patty cakes.

5 Place coconut in plastic bag; tint with yellow colouring. Dip tops
   of eight patty cakes in coconut; position on number 3 cake to
   form caterpillar body. Position jelly beans for feet.

6 Using scissors, cut mallow bake in half; position on remaining
   patty cake for eyes. Using decorating gel, draw dots on mallow
   bakes for pupils.

7 Cut licorice strap lengthways into three strips; tie a knot in the
   end of two of the strips and position on patty cake for antennae.
   Trim remaining strip and position to form mouth; discard remaining
   licorice strip.

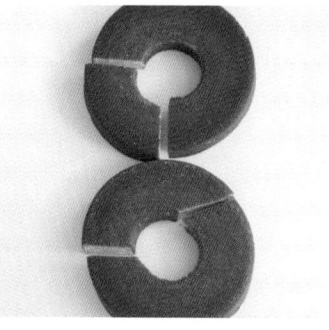

Position the ring cakes cut-side
down. Cut segments out of the
ring cakes, as shown.

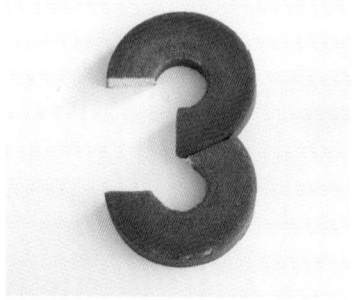

Assemble the cake pieces on
board to form number; discard
remaining pieces.

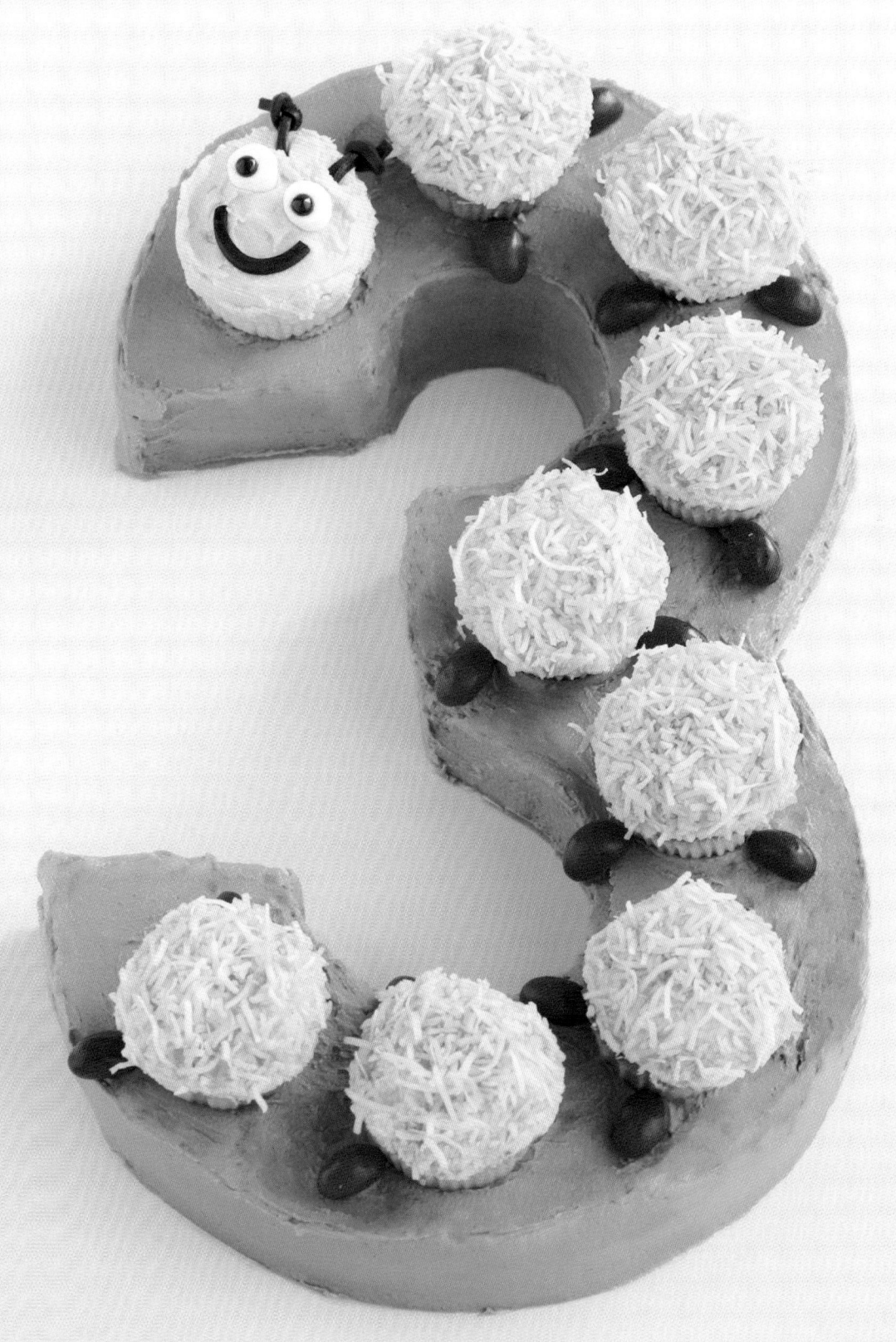

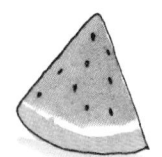 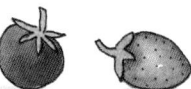

BACON RASHERS also known as slices of bacon, made from pork side, cured and smoked. Middle rashers are the familiar bacon shape, ie, a thin strip of belly pork having a lean, rather round piece of loin at one end; streaky bacon is the same cut minus the round loin section.

BAKING POWDER a raising agent consisting mainly of two parts cream of tartar to one part bicarbonate of soda (baking soda).

BEAN SPROUTS also known as bean shoots; tender new growths of assorted beans and seeds germinated for consumption as sprouts.

BEANS

borlotti also known as roman beans, they can be eaten fresh or dried. Borlotti can also substitute for pinto beans because of the similarity in appearance – both are pale pink or beige with darker red spots.

kidney medium-size red bean, slightly floury yet sweet in flavour; sold dried or canned.

BICARBONATE OF SODA also known as baking soda.

BOK CHOY also known as bak choy, pak choi, chinese white cabbage or chinese chard; has a fresh, mild mustard taste. Use stems and leaves, stir-fried or braised. Baby bok choy, also known as pak kat farang or shanghai bok choy, is smaller and more tender than bok choy.

BREADCRUMBS

packaged fine-textured, crunchy, purchased, white breadcrumbs.

stale one- or two-day-old bread made into crumbs by grating, blending or processing.

BUTTERCAKE MIX packaged cake mix; substitute vanilla, white or yellow cake mixes if you can't find buttercake.

CACHOUS small, round, cake-decorating sweets available in many colours.

CAPSICUM also known as bell pepper or, simply, pepper. Native to Central and South America, they can be red, green, yellow, orange or purplish black. Discard membranes and seeds before use.

CHEESE

bocconcini a walnut-sized, baby mozzarella; delicate, semi-soft, white cheese traditionally made in Italy from buffalo milk. Spoils rapidly so must be kept under refrigeration, in brine, for one or two days at most.

pizza commercial blend comprised of varying proportions of processed grated mozzarella, cheddar and parmesan.

swiss generic name for a variety of cheeses, all of which originate in Switzerland, among them emmentaler and gruyère.

CHICKPEAS also called garbanzos, hummus or channa; an irregularly round, sandy-coloured legume used extensively in Mediterranean and Latin cooking.

CHINESE CABBAGE also known as peking or napa cabbage, wong bok or petsai. Elongated in shape with pale green, crinkly leaves, this is the most common cabbage in South-East Asia. Can be shredded or chopped and eaten raw or braised, steamed or stir-fried.

CHIVES herb related to the onion and leek, with subtle onion flavour. Garlic chives, also known as chinese chives, are strongly flavoured, have flat leaves and are eaten as a vegetable, usually in stir-fries.

COCO POPS chocolate-flavoured puffed rice.

COCONUT

desiccated unsweetened, dried, concentrated, finely shredded coconut.

shredded thin strips of dried coconut.

CORIANDER also known as dhania, cilantro or chinese parsley; bright-green, leafy herb with a pungent flavour used most frequently in the cuisines of Mexico, India and South-East Asia. Often stirred into or sprinkled over a dish just before serving for maximum impact; both the stems and roots of coriander are also used in many Asian dishes.

CORNFLOUR also known as cornstarch; used as a thickening agent in cooking.

COUSCOUS a fine, grain-like cereal product, originally from North Africa; made from semolina.

CRAISINS dried cranberries.

CUMIN also known as zeera, available in ground or seed form; can be purchased from supermarkets.

CUSTARD APPLE also known as cherimoya; a large tropical fruit with pale-green skin and luscious, sweet, white flesh that tastes like a combination of mango, papaya and banana.

CUSTARD POWDER instant mixture used to make pouring custard; similar to North American instant pudding mixes.

FLOUR

plain an all-purpose flour, made from wheat.

FRENCH-TRIMMED LAMB SHANKS also known as drumsticks or Frenched shanks; all the gristle and narrow end of the bone is discarded then the remaining meat trimmed.

HERBS 1 teaspoon dried herbs equals 4 teaspoons (1 tablespoon) chopped fresh herbs.

KUMARA Polynesian name of orange-fleshed sweet potato often confused with yam.

LAVASH unleavened, flat bread originally from the Mediterranean region.

MALLOW BAKES tiny marshmallow squares that come in various flavours used in baking or dessert-making. Sold in 100g cellophane packages.

MANDARIN also known as tangerine; small, loose-skinned citrus fruit that segments easily. Sweeter than an orange, and smaller, but otherwise somewhat similar in appearance.

MELTS

white chocolate discs of compounded white chocolate ideal for melting or moulding.

dark chocolate discs of compounded dark chocolate ideal for melting and moulding.

MINCE (MEAT) ground meat, as in ground beef, ground pork, etc.

MUESLI also known as granola, a combination of grains (mainly oats), nuts and dried fruits. Some manufacturers toast their product in oil and honey, adding crispness and kilojoules.

MUSHROOMS

button small, cultivated white mushrooms with a mild flavour.

enoki long, thin, white mushrooms, with a delicate fruit flavour.

oyster also known as abalone; grey-white mushroom shaped like a fan. Prized for their smooth texture and subtle, oyster-like flavour.

NOODLES

fried crunchy noodles crisp egg noodles sold in packages (commonly a 100g packet), already deep-fried.

hokkien also known as stir-fry noodles; fresh wheat noodles resembling thick, yellow-brown spaghetti needing no pre-cooking before being used.

PATTY-PAN CASES also known as cupcake cakes; accordion-pleated paper or foil lines to fit in the holes of patty-pans, as well as muffin and cupcake moulds.

PATTY PAN SQUASH also known as custard marrow or crookneck pumpkins; a round, slightly flat summer squash being yellow to pale green in colour and having a scalloped edge.

PIE APPLE canned cooked chunky apple used for making pies, muffins etc. Contains no added sugar.

POLENTA also known as cornmeal; a flour-like cereal made of dried corn (maize) sold ground in several different textures; also the name of the dish made from it.

PRAWNS also known as shrimp. There are many species of prawns, the most well known being school, tiger, king and banana.

PRUNES commercially- or sun-dried plums.

RICE

arborio small, round-grain rice well suited to absorb a large amount of liquid; especially suitable for risottos.

basmati a fragrant, white long-grain rice. It should be washed several times prior to cooking.

RICE PAPER SHEETS made from rice paste and stamped into rounds; they store well at room temperature. They're quite brittle and will break if dropped.

RICE BUBBLES puffed rice product made with malt extract, which contains gluten.

RISONI small rice-shape pasta; very similar to another small pasta, orzo.

ROCKET also known as arugula, rugula and rucola; a peppery-tasting green leaf which can be used similarly to baby spinach leaves, eaten raw in salad or used in cooking. Baby rocket leaves are both smaller and less peppery.

ROCKMELON also known as cantaloupe or muskmelon; a large, round fruit with a rough net-like skin and pale orange, soft, perfumed inner flesh.

SAUCES

fish called nam pla on the label if it is Thai made; the Vietnamese version, nuoc nam, is almost identical. Made from pulverised, salted, fermented fish (most often anchovies); has a pungent smell and strong taste.

hoisin a thick, sweet and spicy Chinese paste made from salted fermented soy beans, onions and garlic; used as a marinade or baste, or to accent stir-fries and barbecued or roasted foods.

oyster Asian in origin, this rich, brown sauce is made from oysters and their brine, cooked with salt and soy sauce, and thickened with starches.

tomato pasta sauce, bottled prepared sauce available from supermarkets; sometimes labelled sugo.

STOCK 1 cup (250ml) stock is the equivalent of 1 cup (250ml) water plus 1 crumbled stock cube (or 1 teaspoon stock powder).

SUGAR we used coarse, granulated table sugar, also known as crystal sugar, unless otherwise specified.

brown an extremely soft, finely granulated sugar retaining molasses for its characteristic colour and flavour.

caster also known as superfine or finely granulated table sugar.

icing mixture also known as confectioners' sugar or powdered sugar; pulverised, granulated sugar crushed together with a small amount (about 3%) of cornflour added.

SULTANAS a type of raisin dried from a seedless yellow-green grape of the same name; slightly sweeter and softer than other raisin varieties.

THYME a herb widely used in Mediterranean countries to flavour meats and sauces. Has tiny grey-green leaves that give off a minty, light-lemon aroma.

TOFU also known as bean curd, an off-white, custard-like product made from the "milk" of crushed soy beans; comes fresh as soft or firm, and processed as fried or pressed dried sheets. Leftover fresh tofu can be refrigerated in water (which is changed daily) up to 4 days.

firm made by compressing bean curd to remove most of the water. Good used in stir-fries because it can be tossed without falling apart.

silken refers to the manufacturing method of straining the soy bean liquid through silk.

TORTILLA thin, round unleavened bread originating in Mexico; can be made at home or purchased frozen, fresh or vacuum-packed. Two kinds are available, one made from wheat flour and the other from corn.

VANILLA EXTRACT obtained from vanilla beans infused in water.

WORCESTERSHIRE SAUCE a thin, dark-brown spicy sauce used as a seasoning for meat, gravies and cocktails, and as a condiment.

ZUCCHINI also known as courgette; a small green or yellow member of the squash family having edible flowers.

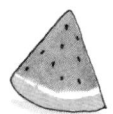

index

facts + figures

Wherever you live, you'll be able to use our recipes with the help of these easy-to-follow conversions. While these conversions are approximate only, the difference between an exact and the approximate conversion of various liquid and dry measures is minimal and will not affect your cooking results.

LIQUID MEASURES

METRIC	IMPERIAL
30ml	1 fluid oz
60ml	2 fluid oz
100ml	3 fluid oz
125ml	4 fluid oz
150ml	5 fluid oz (¼ pint/1 gill)
190ml	6 fluid oz
250ml	8 fluid oz
300ml	10 fluid oz (½ pint)
500ml	16 fluid oz
600ml	20 fluid oz (1 pint)
1000ml (1 litre)	1¾ pints

DRY MEASURES

METRIC	IMPERIAL
15g	½oz
30g	1oz
60g	2oz
90g	3oz
125g	4oz (¼lb)
155g	5oz
185g	6oz
220g	7oz
250g	8oz (½lb)
280g	9oz
315g	10oz
345g	11oz
375g	12oz (¾lb)
410g	13oz
440g	14oz
470g	15oz
500g	16oz (1lb)
750g	24oz (1½lb)
1kg	32oz (2lb)

HELPFUL MEASURES

METRIC	IMPERIAL
3mm	⅛in
6mm	¼in
1cm	½in
2cm	¾in
2.5cm	1in
5cm	2in
6cm	2½in
8cm	3in
10cm	4in
13cm	5in
15cm	6in
18cm	7in
20cm	8in
23cm	9in
25cm	10in
28cm	11in
30cm	12in (1ft)

MEASURING EQUIPMENT

The difference between one country's measuring cups and another's is, at most, within a 2 or 3 teaspoon variance. (For the record, one Australian metric measuring cup holds approximately 250ml.) The most accurate way of measuring dry ingredients is to weigh them. When measuring liquids, use a clear glass or plastic jug with metric markings. (One Australian metric tablespoon holds 20ml; one Australian metric teaspoon holds 5ml.)

HOW TO MEASURE

When using graduated metric measuring cups, shake dry ingredients loosely into the appropriate cup. Do not tap the cup on a bench or tightly pack the ingredients unless directed to do so. Level top of measuring cups and measuring spoons with a knife. When measuring liquids, place a clear glass or plastic jug with metric markings on a flat surface to check accuracy at eye level.

Note: North America, NZ and the UK use 15ml tablespoons. All cup and spoon measurements are level.

We use large eggs having an average weight of 60g.

OVEN TEMPERATURES

These oven temperatures are only a guide. Always check the manufacturer's manual.

	°C (CELSIUS)	°F (FAHRENHEIT)	GAS MARK
Very slow	120	250	½
Slow	140-150	275-300	1-2
Moderately slow	170	325	3
Moderate	180-190	350-375	4-5
Moderately hot	200	400	6
Hot	220-230	425-450	7-8
Very hot	240	475	9

ARE YOU MISSING SOME OF THE WORLD'S FAVOURITE COOKBOOKS?

The Australian Women's Weekly Cookbooks are available from bookshops, cookshops, supermarkets and other stores all over the world. You can also buy direct from the publisher, using the order form below.

TITLE	RRP	QTY	TITLE	RRP	QTY
Almost Vegetarian	£5.99		Good Food Fast	£5.99	
Asian, Meals in Minutes	£5.99		Great Lamb Cookbook	£5.99	
Babies & Toddlers Good Food	£5.99		Greek Cooking Class	£5.99	
Barbecue Meals In Minutes	£5.99		Healthy Heart Cookbook	£5.99	
Basic Cooking Class	£5.99		Indian Cooking Class	£5.99	
Beginners Cooking Class	£5.99		Japanese Cooking Class	£5.99	
Beginners Simple Meals	£5.99		Kids' Birthday Cakes	£5.99	
Beginners Thai	£5.99		Kids Cooking	£5.99	
Best Ever Slimmers' Recipes	£5.99		Lean Food	£5.99	
Best Food	£5.99		Low-carb, Low-fat	£5.99	
Best Food Desserts	£5.99		Low-fat Feasts	£5.99	
Best Food Fast	£5.99		Low-fat Food For Life	£5.99	
Best Food Mains	£5.99		Low-fat Meals in Minutes	£5.99	
Cakes Cooking Class	£5.99		Main Course Salads	£5.99	
Caribbean Cooking	£5.99		Middle Eastern Cooking Class	£5.99	
Casseroles	£5.99		Midweek Meals in Minutes	£5.99	
Chicken Meals in Minutes	£5.99		Muffins, Scones & Bread	£5.99	
Chinese Cooking Class	£5.99		New Casseroles	£5.99	
Christmas Cooking	£5.99		New Classics	£5.99	
Cocktails	£5.99		New Finger Food	£5.99	
Cooking for Friends	£5.99		Party Food and Drink (Oct 05)	£5.99	
Creative Cooking on a Budget	£5.99		Pasta Meals in Minutes	£5.99	
Detox (Sept 05)	£5.99		Potatoes	£5.99	
Dinner Beef	£5.99		Quick Meals in Minutes	£5.99	
Dinner Lamb (Aug 05)	£5.99		Salads: Simple, Fast & Fresh	£5.99	
Dinner Seafood	£5.99		Saucery	£5.99	
Easy Australian Style	£5.99		Sensational Stir-Fries	£5.99	
Easy Curry	£5.99		Short-order Cook	£5.99	
Easy Spanish-Style	£5.99		Slim	£5.99	
Essential Soup	£5.99		Sweet Old Fashioned Favourites	£5.99	
Freezer, Meals from the	£5.99		Thai Cooking Class	£5.99	
French Cooking Class	£5.99		Vegetarian Meals in Minutes	£5.99	
French Food, New	£5.99		Weekend Cook	£5.99	
Fresh Food for Babies & Toddlers	£5.99		Wicked Sweet Indulgences	£5.99	
Get Real, Make a Meal	£5.99		Wok, Meals in Minutes	£5.99	
			TOTAL COST:	**£**	

NAME

ADDRESS

POSTCODE

DAYTIME PHONE

I ENCLOSE MY CHEQUE/MONEY ORDER FOR £

OR PLEASE CHARGE MY VISA, ACCESS OR MASTERCARD NUMBER

CARD HOLDER'S NAME

EXPIRY DATE

CARDHOLDER'S SIGNATURE

To order: Mail or fax – photocopy or complete the order form above, and send your credit card details or cheque payable to: Australian Consolidated Press (UK), Moulton Park Business Centre, Red House Road, Moulton Park, Northampton NN3 6AQ, phone (+44) (0) 1604 497531, fax (+44) (0) 1604 497533, e-mail books@acpuk.com Or order online at www.acpuk.com

Non-UK residents: We accept the credit cards listed on the coupon, or cheques, drafts or International Money Orders payable in sterling and drawn on a UK bank. Credit card charges are at the exchange rate current at the time of payment.

Postage and packing UK: Add £1.00 per order plus 50p per book.

Postage and packing overseas: Add £2.00 per order plus £1.00 per book.

Offer ends 31.12.2006

Test Kitchen
Food director *Pamela Clark*
Food editor *Karen Hammial*
Assistant food editor *Amira Georgy*
Test Kitchen manager *Cathie Lonnie*
Home economists *Sammie Coryton, Nancy Duran, Nicole Jennings, Elizabeth Macri, Christina Martignago, Sharon Reeve, Susie Riggall, Kirrily Smith*
Editorial coordinator *Rebecca Steyns*

ACP Books
Editorial director *Susan Tomnay*
Creative director *Hieu Chi Nguyen*
Feature writer and senior editor *Julie Collard*
Designers *Corey Butler, Lena Lowe*
Consultant dietitian *Susan Thompson*
Illustrations *Louise Pfanner*
Studio manager *Caryl Wiggins*
Design assistant *Josii Do*
Editorial coordinator *Merryn Pearse*
Sales director *Brian Cearnes*
Rights manager *Jane Hazell*
Marketing director *Matt Dominello*
Brand manager *Renée Crea*
Sales and marketing coordinator *Gabrielle Botto*
Manager demand planning *Daniel Prasad*
Pre-press *Harry Palmer*
Production manager *Carol Currie*
Business manager *Seymour Cohen*
Business analyst *Marena Paul*
Chief executive officer *John Alexander*
Group publisher *Pat Ingram*
Publisher *Sue Wannan*
Editor-in-chief *Deborah Thomas*

Produced by ACP Books, Sydney.
Printed by Times Printers, Singapore.
Published by ACP Publishing Pty Limited, 54 Park St, Sydney; GPO Box 4088, Sydney, NSW 2001.
Ph: (02) 9282 8618 Fax: (02) 9267 9438.
acpbooks@acp.com.au
www.acpbooks.com.au
To order books, phone 136 116.
Send recipe enquiries to:
recipeenquiries@acp.com.au

RIGHTS ENQUIRIES
Laura Bamford, Director ACP Books.
lbamford@acplon.co.uk
Ph: +44 (207) 812 6526
AUSTRALIA: Distributed by Network Services, GPO Box 4088, Sydney, NSW 2001.
Ph: (02) 9282 8777 Fax: (02) 9264 3278.
UNITED KINGDOM: Distributed by Australian Consolidated Press (UK), Moulton Park Business Centre, Red House Rd, Moulton Park, Northampton, NN3 6AQ.
Ph: (01604) 497531 Fax: (01604) 497533
acpukltd@aol.com
CANADA: Distributed by Whitecap Books Ltd, 351 Lynn Ave, North Vancouver, BC, V7J 2C4.
Ph: (604) 980 9852 Fax: (604) 980 8197
customerservice@whitecap.ca
www.whitecap.ca
NEW ZEALAND: Distributed by Netlink Distribution Company, ACP Media Centre, Cnr Fanshawe and Beaumont Streets, Westhaven, Auckland.
PO Box 47906, Ponsonby, Auckland, NZ.
Ph: (09) 366 9966 ask@ndcnz.co.nz
SOUTH AFRICA: Distributed by PSD Promotions, 30 Diesel Road Isando, Gauteng Johannesburg.
PO Box 1175, Isando 1600, Gauteng Johannesburg.
Ph: (2711) 392 6065/6/7
Fax: (2711) 392 6079/80
orders@psdprom.co.za

Clark, Pamela.
The Australian Women's Weekly
Fresh food for babies & toddlers.

Includes index.
ISBN 186396 415 0
1. Cookery (Baby foods). 2. Infants – nutrition.
I. Title. II. Title: Australian Women's Weekly.

641.56222

© ACP Publishing Pty Limited 2005
ABN 18 053 273 546
This publication is copyright. No part of it may be reproduced or transmitted in any form without the written permission of the publishers.

The publishers would like to thank the following for props used in photography:
Duck Egg Blue; Honeybee Homewares; Iced Affair Cake Decorating; IKEA; Queen Bee Balloon and Party Shop; The Essential Ingredient; Villeroy & Boch.